Be
POWERFUL

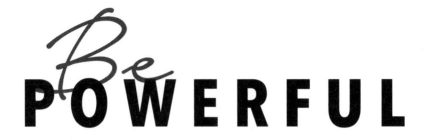

Be POWERFUL

FIND YOUR
STRENGTH
AT ANY AGE

LIZ HILLIARD

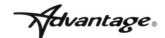

Published by Advantage, Charleston, South Carolina.
Member of Advantage Media Group.

ADVANTAGE is a registered trademark, and the Advantage colophon is a trademark of Advantage Media Group, Inc.

Printed in the United States of America.

ISBN: 978-1-59932-743-3
LCCN: 2016955469

Cover design by Katie Biondo.

This publication is designed to provide accurate and authoritative information in regard to the subject matter covered. It is sold with the understanding that the publisher is not engaged in rendering legal, accounting, or other professional services. If legal advice or other expert assistance is required, the services of a competent professional person should be sought.

Advantage Media Group is proud to be a part of the Tree Neutral® program. Tree Neutral offsets the number of trees consumed in the production and printing of this book by taking proactive steps such as planting trees in direct proportion to the number of trees used to print books. To learn more about Tree Neutral, please visit **www.treeneutral.com.**

TreeNeutral

Advantage Media Group is a publisher of business, self-improvement, and professional development books. We help entrepreneurs, business leaders, and professionals share their Stories, Passion, and Knowledge to help others Learn & Grow. Do you have a manuscript or book idea that you would like us to consider for publishing? Please visit **advantagefamily.com** or call **1.866.775.1696.**

To Clary, my light and inspiration.

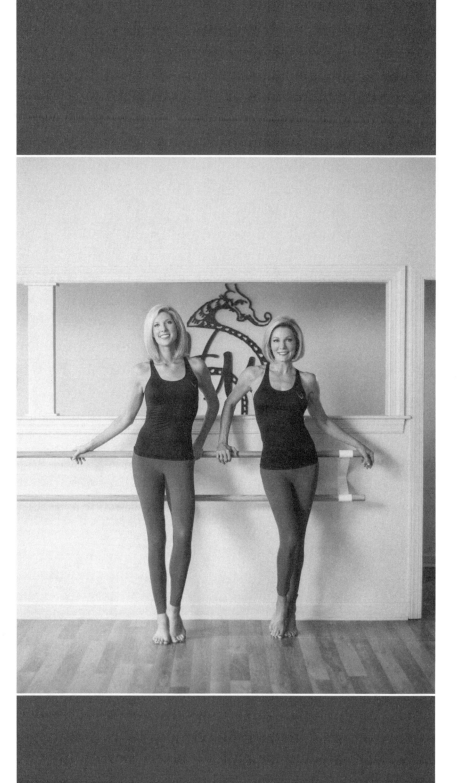

TABLE OF CONTENTS

"The difference between an ordinary man and a warrior is that a warrior takes everything as a challenge while an ordinary man takes everything as a blessing or a curse."

—Carlos Castaneda, *The Tales of Power*

I believe we all have the extraordinary strength of a warrior inside us that is ready to spring to life in overwhelming circumstances. This book is about my own story of tapping into my power and how, through physical exercise and will, I learned the means needed to overcome many of life's obstacles. I invite you to come with me on this journey to find your strengths. To find your strength is to know your weakness, acknowledge and embrace it, and then find your joy, which is your most authentic self. I believe that living joyfully is our most natural state, and all the rest is an illusion.

Hilliard Studio Method was born as an answer to my daughter's request to be in the best shape of her life for her wedding. Little did I know how powerful that request would be, not only for the two of us as mother and daughter but also for our clients. Whether it's your first or fiftieth class, our workout will possibly be the toughest physical challenge of your day and, in equal measure, a joy of accomplishment and strength that will last you all day.

The story of Hilliard Studio Method begins with my own journey through darkness and how I found a way to embrace my power and find my authentic self, which is joy. That joy existed when

I was a child, but I began to understand it more powerfully the day my daughter, Clary, was born. I remember looking down at her and thinking, *Oh, it's you!* with a sense of recognition and relief.

Our lives became entwined from day one. She was born my best friend, and as best friends, we were almost never apart. Clary came with me everywhere, even to the modeling shoots and fashion shows that I did when she was quite young, even snagging her first paying job when she was nine making $30 an hour as my dresser for shows! We traveled together, explored together, and found magic together wherever we were. And whatever it was we wound up doing, I made sure even the smallest things were an adventure. Life, I told her, is about joy. And she was my joy! I told her that as often as I could.

Even now, in our "big girl" jobs—for me as the CEO of Hilliard Studio Method, and for Clary, as the director of marketing—at the end of the day, the most important part of our business is the strength of our relationship and our *joie de vivre*. The concept of living joyfully in the face of any circumstance is my philosophy. Our joy exists in our love and respect for each other, so planning and creating together flows naturally. Ours is a symbiotic relationship in which we both feel independent and able to bring our different strengths to the table and also one in which we have learned how to support each other in our weaknesses. We work hard and we have fun, and I honestly can't imagine doing this job and taking this journey without Clary. She is, after all, the reason Hilliard Studio Method exists in the first place.

I am fortunate to have given birth to my greatest friend and perfect business partner and feel fortunate to own a successful and growing business, but in the end, the fact is we make our own fortune. It doesn't always come easily, of course, and I have learned that failure is not fatal, and success is not final. To recognize the bad times with the good times and understand that neither defines us is powerful.

What defines us is how we react and behave through both the bad and good times. That understanding—knowing that you stand in the middle and deciding which side you'll embrace—is when you learn who you truly are.

Failure is not fatal, and success is not final.

This book is about embracing your own strength and power in order to find your authentic self and live life to its fullest. To know your strengths—physical, mental, and emotional—you must first know and acknowledge your weakness. This book begins with my own journey and how I found my power, but it will become about you and your journey in finding your strength to discover your own power and joy amid the chaos of life. Your power already exists in you. I recognize that it takes power to make fitness and health a priority. It takes power to push your body to the place where it will change. It takes power to embrace your authentic self. That power already exists within each of us, but at Hilliard Studio Method we remind you that it is already there.

1

GOING THROUGH HELL
IN GASOLINE DRAWERS

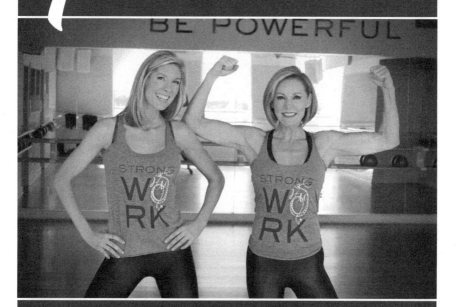

CHAPTER 1:
GOING THROUGH HELL IN GASOLINE DRAWERS

*Power begins by finding your authentic self, embracing it, and then releasing it into the world around you. Power is your absolute knowledge, love, and acceptance of yourself, and it comes from knowing **who** you are, not what you know. Regardless of whatever turns your life may take, this power exists in all of us.*

The story of Hilliard Studio Method begins with my own journey through self-doubt and darkness and how I found a way to embrace my authentic self and find my power. It was an awakening that happened in many stages and on many levels, culminating in an understanding of my own strength and the knowledge that *I am worthy* simply because I believe I am, despite what I may have been told or believed in the past.

When we're young, we're shaped in large part by the world around us and by what others believe, whether it's through what we're told, how we're treated, or what people expect of us. Those beliefs of childhood often linger well into our adult years, so it becomes important to address them, carefully weighing whether or not they still serve us and taking into consideration how we react to them as we grow older. If, for example, we were led to believe that we were not good enough as children, as adults, we now have the choice to continue that belief or choose otherwise.

MY MOST POWERFUL TEACHER

I was eight years old the first time I was told I was stupid. I was born in 1954 to two very intellectual parents. My sister, Wallis, was thirteen when I came along and was like a protective mother to me. Not only was she sweet and loving, she was incredibly smart and attended Duke University on full academic scholarship. My brother, Pete, was five years older than me and just as smart as Wallis. He and I were close and insanely competitive.

Our family dinner table was where I received my education. By the time I was going through school, my parents were exhausted, and I was expected to do more on my own. There wasn't much emphasis on my schoolwork, and when I was in school I was bored and resentful of having to sit still all day between what seemed like four heavy, dark walls.

When we were all together, my family vigorously debated about current events, history, and philosophy, and we agreed and disagreed with a great sense of passion and respect for each other's opinions. As the littlest one at the table, I just tried to keep up with the conversation and not miss the food as it was passed around. My sister dubbed me "the human sponge" since I would listen, soak up, and reiterate the things they were saying. We had no fear about speaking our minds. We were allowed to think outside the box, which was a rare and powerful gift given to us by our parents. Fear wasn't a way for us. Old or young, male or female, we were taught to stand up for ourselves and for what we believed.

I felt worthy and accepted at home, and I had a natural sense of happiness, joy, and confidence. As a very young girl, I remember jumping on my mom and dad's bed early every morning, waking them up to the sound of my favorite chant, "I am the spirit of Liz, made like a whiz!" I doubt that it was their favorite chant! From dawn to dusk, I would run with my brother and his friends. They treated me as one of the boys and were definitely not afraid to include me in their games and roughhousing, and it was during these days of splashing in the creek and racing through the neighborhood that I developed such an intense competitive drive and a love for freedom and movement.

But I'll never forget that when I was eight years old, my third grade teacher told me I was stupid and would never see the fourth grade. She was a frightening woman with netted, blue hair and gnarled, witchy hands. Every day, she would line us up at the door for a parting word, and every day, she rapped my hands with a wooden ruler, driving into my head and my heart that I was stupid. It was humiliating, hurtful, and unfortunately quite powerful.

She was the meanest woman I had ever met, but she taught me the power that a person you respect, whether out of fear or out of love, can have on your life. It was because of this difficult lesson—that we can either strip the power from one another or we can empower one another—that I call her my greatest teacher.

She may have planted the seed for my academic self-doubt, but through elementary, middle, and high school I excelled as an athlete and had plenty of friends who helped me overcome the feeling of being stupid. Movement played a key role in helping me find my strength and inner joy. I was especially passionate about basketball and was the leading scorer for my high school, earning all-conference titles for three years straight. Driven by a competitive will, I had found my place to excel both on the court and off as the chief majorette. I choreographed routines of precision, flow, and energy, likely influencing the way I began to weave together the movements used for Hilliard Studio Method as much as my Pilates training did.

During my senior year of high school, I was called into a conference with my psychology teacher. I was doing reasonably well in her class and genuinely respected her. I remember yearning for a pep-talk type of conversation that sounded something like "Liz, you're doing a great job in my class this year, and I feel you've been underestimating yourself," but instead, I was blindsided and further defeated by

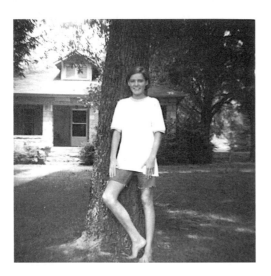

her blunt explanation that I should probably consider other options besides going to college. I did, in fact, get accepted to Elon University, but with low academic self-worth and a keen ability to party, I ended up, after two years, at a local community college, which for me was the ultimate confirmation that I was actually stupid. I was living at home while getting a community college associate degree in dental hygiene, and even though I made straight As and did well, I couldn't shake the lingering feelings of self-doubt.

Despite believing I was stupid, I maintained an intense inner sense of joy that did not bow to criticism and refused to be silenced. It was my conviction that, deep down, I felt peace and comfort in understanding I was in some way more than what I was being told.

That joy persevered throughout my life with no rhyme or reason in the face of every circumstance. I now recognize that joy as my truest self, my authentic self.

I AM WORTHY

The first time I experienced devastating pain and loss was when my father suddenly died of a heart attack when I was sixteen years old. Losing a parent or loved one at any age is difficult, but as an emotional teenager, I remember feeling somehow guilty about his death. I wondered what I could have done differently to keep him alive. I lost him at a time when I probably needed a strong, male influence in my life to model the type of man I should choose for myself. And until I met my husband, I didn't make very good choices about boyfriends.

No one told me I was worthy. Just me. That inner joy, that strength, my authentic self, refused to be quiet another moment, and I proved that to myself when I most needed to walk away from a bad relationship. While I was in dental-hygiene school, I became engaged and started living with a recently divorced dentist who turned out to be rolling through the 1970s in a drug-induced haze. It was one night when he was having a brief phone call with his four-year-old daughter that I knew I needed to walk away and not look back. As I listened to him slurring, unable to get his words out coherently, I could hear his daughter crying "Daddy!" on the other end of the line. The pain in her voice was devastating to me. In that moment it became crystal clear that this was not a life I wanted any part of. I simply walked out, left everything behind, and wrote myself a letter that read, "I am worthy. I am better than this."

On that day I decided once and for all that *I was enough!* So I walked away.

Years later, after Hilliard Studio Method was in full swing, I was reminded of that moment when I received a note from one of my clients.

11

During a recent class, I'd referred to our back muscles as our "walking-away muscles."

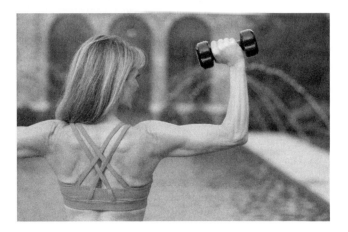

"This might be the day you need to walk away from something, so you might as well look good doing it!" I said, not knowing the incredible impact those words would have.

A few days later I was touched to receive this letter:

March 28, 2014

Dear Liz,

I just wanted to share a little personal moment with you. Let me first say I am totally and completely addicted to the workout you have created. It is like none other! I feel stronger every day!

But the emotional benefits were crystallized for me yesterday.

During your class, you made a comment during our back/upper-body exercises, that "someday you might have to walk away, and you want to look smokin' hot from behind" or something like that ...and it resonated with me, because I have been off-and-on lately with a bad relationship that I just didn't feel strong enough to walk away from! And I feel so much stronger today as a result! And I just wanted to say thank you!

Sincerely,

Heather McNaull, age 41

Heather's heart-spoken words only reinforced in me the realization that we truly never know how the truth we speak will inspire or cause a turning point in someone's life.

To be able to cast aside the voices in us that tell us we are not worthy is powerful. Realizing that we have the power to define our own self-worth and not let others steal our joy is courageous and a necessary step in becoming powerful.

FINDING MY INNER STRENGTH

By 1980, I'd graduated from college and was living comfortably with a good job in dental hygiene when I met and married my husband, Aubrey. Within eight months of our love-at-first-sight meeting we were married, and our long-lasting love has grown from our breathless courtship to a lifetime of love and respect. In 1982 when our daughter Clary was born, it seemed everything, finally, was the way it should be. We were happy, and those old feelings of stupidity and unworthiness became buried in joy.

But at some point, or at many different points in our lives, we go through dark, sad, or challenging times in some form. Whether we are faced with daily frustrations or long-term problems, personal struggles, or lifetime losses, we all experience the human emotions that can hold us back from recognizing our power. I lost my power more than once.

My husband was in the oil and gas business when the boom that brought us bounty early in the eighties turned into a bust when oil prices fell to historic lows and nearly everyone in that industry went bankrupt. Never in a million years did I think that could happen to us, but in spite of all Aubrey's efforts it did. We were nearly destitute and nearly lost our home and all possessions. These were bleak and lonely times when even those people you thought were your dearest friends shunned you. We found the path back to solvency after several years.

> *"Midway along the journey of our life*
> *I woke to find myself in a dark wood,*
> *for I had wandered off from the straight path.*
> *How hard it is to tell what it was like,*
> *this wood of wilderness, savage and stubborn*
> *(the thought of it brings back all my old fears),*
> *a bitter place! Death could scarce be bitterer.*
> *But if I would show the good that came of it,*
> *I must talk about things other than good."*

> –Dante, *Inferno*

The second significant time I felt stripped of my power was when I happened to be reading a book by Helen Luke, called *Dark Wood to Red Rose: Journey and Transformation in Dante's Divine Comedy*.

In the midst of my "dark wood," I felt paralyzed, as if trapped in ice as Dante described in *Inferno*, and simply could not move. I felt naked, afraid, and exposed and that everything that defined me was in question or simply lost. All I could do was move forward, as movement had always defined me. I choose not to name that time, because to name it would lend it power. And while no one wants to go through hell doused in gasoline, sometimes the fire that feels like it's burning you is actually burning away the weakness and doubt that were holding you back to help you find clarity. When you stand in the midst of the fire and start to breathe through the face of fear, you reclaim yourself and allow your soul to fly.

During this time Clary was fourteen years old, a pivotal time in a girl's life, and my mother was on her deathbed. I wanted to protect my daughter and was terrified to lose my mother, but it was *she* who in her darkest days was trying to empower and comfort *me*. She'd contracted hepatitis C from a blood transfusion at a time before blood screenings were done. It had led to cirrhosis of the liver, and during that time, she kept coming close to death. She was the strongest woman I'd ever known, but her body was failing her.

I remember standing by her bed one day in particular and my whole body was aching. I wasn't sick, but she sensed my fear because she came out of one of those mild coma states she kept slipping into, looked at me, and said, "I want you to stop worrying right now. I'm not going to leave you alone in your darkness." Just those brief words were so empowering. And in lifting me up, I found ways to lift our family up. I told Clary the truth: that life can be hard on us at times and everything you do carries risk. I told her, "We are a family, and we will prevail through any hardship and come out better on the other side. So go to school. Do your work. Play volleyball. I'll be here every day to pick you up."

When my mother did die, Aubrey, Clary, and I had each other, and we were strong again. My mother's enduring gift of love was the most empowering thing she gave me. What I realized without her was that I had to be strong for my family and carry on her legacy of generosity, joy, hard work, and unconditional love. Each day my goal is to live and work that way.

Just by standing and slowly taking steps on the path of the crooked, unknown road, by experiencing the bad and gaining newfound respect for the good, I was able to start to see hope. Each step forward was a step of strength and recognition that I could shape a new path, so I kept putting one foot in front of the other.

But what I learned is that in our darkest moments, when our worst fears have come true and our personal demons have reared their ugly heads, we have two choices: we can choose to stand up, even if it's on wobbly knees, or we can give up. The choice to take a breath is powerful. The choice to stand in the face of fear is powerful, and the choice to stand on your own in the midst of powerlessness and hopelessness is heroic.

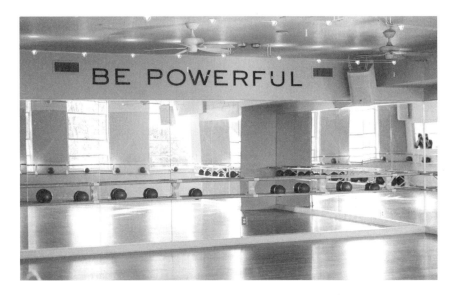

BE POWERFUL

We all go through dark times, and everyone's experience is different. It doesn't matter what the challenging time is. What's significant is that in that moment, in that time of helplessness, you feel powerless. You never know who is standing in front of you, scared to death and living in the midst of his or her own personal hell. While teaching my classes, I see the faces of the clients in the room and, sometimes, sense their need to feel they can accomplish something—anything— not just the exercise but also some proof of their strength; they need to see how *powerful* they really are.

"Be Powerful" is my mantra. It is written across the wall at Hilliard Studio Method. We meet our clients wherever they are and show them how powerful they can be even in the face of adversity. I can look at a client and say, "Look at you! Look at what you just did!" I point to them across a full classroom and say, "Do you see you? Look in the mirror and look at you. See how powerful you are."

What matters in that moment is that they realize how strong they *can be*. If they've never done a bicep curl or a push-up in their lives, it doesn't matter. After confronting my own fears, it's my joy to help others with a kind word or an extra push-up to do the same. It's not about perfection; it's about giving it a shot and reaching beyond your perceived boundaries. When you reach your edge physically or emotionally, it's that extra effort that makes the change and empowers you in all areas of your life. That's power.

When I created Hilliard Studio Method, I knew I wanted to teach people that physical power could change their lives and have an impact not only on them physically but mentally and emotionally as well. We've created a community

> When you reach your edge physically or emotionally, it's that extra effort that makes the change and empowers you in all areas of your life. That's power.

of support and encouragement to help you through your physical and mental barriers, enabling you to find your strongest and most powerful self. That power teaches you that when you put your head and heart into something, you are unstoppable. That's why Hilliard Studio Method works. It pushes you to the edge and transforms your body and your mind.

*S*weating, swearing, and shocked—that is how I ended my very first class at Hilliard Studio Method. As a lifelong athlete and professional swimmer, I seldom come up against a physical challenge that I cannot figure out and eventually grasp. The Hilliard Studio Method Amazons (Liz and Clary) made quick work of my theory. Intrigued and determined to master the dreaded "pretzel," I returned for more. Some moves I rocked (overhead shoulder press, yes) and some moves rocked *me* (hello, thighs). *This can't be happening*, I thought, incredulous that I could no longer pulse in a "Friday-night high-heel," while the trainers strongly encouraged another twenty.

What kept me coming back to class was, and still is, the challenge for ego and my mental toughness. Slowly, one pelvic tilt at a time, I have come to realize the greatest gift Hilliard Studio Method has given me: *power*. I have the power to push my mind and body to failure so that I may gain strength. Now, I see the times that I must lower my heels or rest my arms as a training tool that will not only boost but also catapult me to the next level.

I have made a career out of finding and embracing that break-through feeling, and I am thrilled to have found a beautiful environment for me to cultivate that feeling consistently.

–MADISON KENNEDY, HILLIARD STUDIO METHOD TRAINER, AGE 28

PROFESSIONAL SWIMMER, 4X50 SCM FREESTYLE WORLD RECORD, 3RD PLACE FINISH AT THE 2016 USA OLYMPIC TRIALS

2

TORONTO, A WEDDING, AND THE METHOD

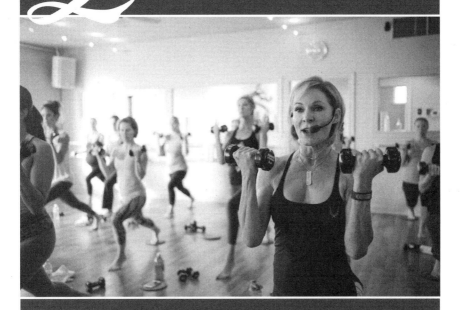

CHAPTER 2:
TORONTO, A WEDDING, AND THE METHOD

I still remember the look on my husband's face when I told him that I would be going to Toronto for ten weeks to become a Pilates instructor at the cost of $5,000, not including room and board.

Our only child had just left for college, and now I was planning to leave to pursue a brand-new dream. I had fallen in love with Pilates after taking my first class in Charlotte in 1999. It was the physical challenge I had been missing in my life, and getting my ass kicked had triggered my competitive spirit. Other exercise classes generally bored me to death, but this kept my attention.

My instructor in that first class became my first Pilates personal trainer, a good friend, and eventually, my business associate. She trained me in a small studio that happens to be a stone's throw away from what was to become our flagship Hilliard Studio Method Charlotte, North Carolina, location.

After just a few months, my new passion for Pilates led me to explore the possibility of becoming a Pilates-certified personal trainer. In typical fashion, I wasn't worried about the obstacles, including a pricy and lengthy move to Toronto to train at the STOTT PILATES International Training Institute.

WHAT IS PILATES?

Pilates Is a core-centric workout developed by the late Joseph Pilates as a means to strengthen the core. That means engaging the muscles of the torso in every movement you do. Pilates works your muscles through stretch with light resistance, promoting a long lean body, flat abdominal muscles, and a strong back.

TRAINING IN TORONTO

I spent most of the summer of 2002, and part of that fall training and becoming certified at STOTT. As long as I live, I'll never forget the first day I walked into class.

There were maybe fifteen other students in the room, and just as we were sitting down, the strong and stoic top trainer walked in, looked right at me, and said, "Name the four abdominal groups and how they work."

I was mortified! We must have been given some assignment to do before the class, but I hadn't done it, so I asked, "Can I get back with you on that?"

The stare-down she gave me said, "Don't ever walk in this studio again unless you know what you're talking about."

She didn't have to ask anyone else that question because, suddenly, everyone in the class was firing off intricately explained answers about muscular anatomy, form, and function.

When I returned to class the next day, I was in a cold sweat. I was mentally begging the instructor not to ask me any particularly hard questions, or for that matter, *any* questions, but when she finally shot one to me, I nailed it.

I was staying for those long ten weeks at a bed-and-breakfast twenty minutes outside of the city where I would stay up late studying and engaging with the owner and her loud-mouth parrot about my training. Aubrey was at home working and Clary was enjoying her first year at UNC-Chapel Hill, and I think they were both wondering if I had lost my mind or was having a midlife crisis! You don't usually move to another country to train for your passion, but I did, and I was going to make every moment worth it.

Our training routine included that daily anatomy quiz, and then we would go into the workout, focusing on one exercise for the entire day. We learned every aspect of the movement and every modification. We learned every detail about which muscles were contracting or extending and abducting and adducting, their connections, and their impact on the movement of the body. At the end of the day, we broke into groups and took turns being the teacher. We practiced instructing each other through the movements and muscle function.

It was intense, difficult, and extremely regimented to say the least. I came away at the end of those ten weeks not only with an incredible knowledge of the human body but also with a highly regarded and hard-earned Pilates certification, ready to make the next step of opening my own Pilates studio.

PERFORMANCE PILATES

My first rent-free studio was a small room in my husband's office. It was a typical office space with a sterile feeling inspired by bad carpeting and fluorescent lighting. I filled my room with three pieces of Pilates equipment and trained clients all day on the hour. My first instinct was to name the business Power Pilates, but that name was taken, so I chose Performance Pilates, which translated well since I wanted to train my clients to *perform* better in their day-to-day lives.

I wanted to teach them how to function properly in their bodies and connect their movements to their breath, all while deeply engaging the core muscles.

I remember being scared to death when my first client walked through the door. Pilates, especially STOTT PILATES, is a take-no-prisoner kind of workout, so you better know your stuff or you'll be weeded out of the business quickly. I had to rely on the fact that I knew what I was doing and was well trained and prepared. It was risky to start my own business, but the reward came quickly in getting to know my clients.

One of the first times I realized I was making a difference was when a client I had been working with for just a couple of months spent our entire one-hour session in tears. The moment she walked in, she sat down, dropped her head and her shoulders, and began to shake. I sat beside her, put my arm around her shoulder, and listened. She confided in me all the things that were currently making her feel weak, scared, and stressed. She trusted me and knew that not only would the things she shared with me be kept private but also that I cared about what she was going through.

My plan for her that day was focused on physical training, but I knew she needed an emotional release that would allow her to feel better when she walked out the door. Looking back, I'm almost positive that every single client I have trained personally had a moment when she just needed to break down and cry. In fact, the business model for Hilliard Studio Method draws, essentially, from directly answering the needs of my clients. It is about empowerment, trust, community, and the recognition that we are all trying our best.

I learned that a personal, emotional connection was what made my sessions more than what you could get at a typical gym or fitness class experience. Not only was I able to provide a physically challenging, effective, and efficient workout, but I was able to form a relationship with my clients that was built on trust and allowed them to make a deeper connection to their overall wellness, not just their physical being. The stronger they felt emotionally—their recognition of their potential power—the stronger they felt physically.

I may not always know the struggles individuals in my class are experiencing, but my goal, as a personal and group trainer, is always to support them in all the different phases of their lives.

> Hilliard Studio Method is about empowerment, trust, community, and the recognition that we are all trying our best.

When I think of Hilliard Studio Method, I think of their positive, youthful energy and encouraging words. There is a reason that their phrase is "Be Powerful." Take one look at Liz and Clary Hilliard Gray and you can immediately tell how healthy and fit they are from the inside out. I wanted that energy! Hilliard Studio Method is much more than an exercise class, as they are promoting and teaching total wellness.

I remember when I first started over a year ago and struggled, Liz and all the instructors would say, "strong work." Those encouraging words resonated with me, as I believe physical strength helps us become stronger emotionally and mentally as well. As one of the "older" ladies there, I know firsthand that life is full of challenges and that women handle many of the bumps in the road for our families, work, and communities, so maintaining and increasing our physical strength is critical for our long-term health and emotional well-being. I just kept showing up and getting stronger week by week.

Since my teens and twenties, I have done weight training, yoga, spin classes, aerobic classes, triathlon training, etc., but Hilliard is one of the most efficient and effective workouts I have tried. I have lost weight, trimmed the muffin top, strengthened my core, which also improved my posture, and sculpted my arms and legs. As we age, strengthening and protecting our joints becomes much more important as well, and I feel Hilliard Studio Method has also helped my joints. Though I thought I knew a lot about nutrition, I have also learned fresh ideas for improving the way I fuel my body. I recently went snow skiing and felt great!

The investment of time and money in attending classes at Hilliard Studio Method is one of the wisest I have made in years! We need to care for ourselves as we care for our families, work, and communities. We truly can be younger next year, and Liz is living proof.

–CAROL ROBINSON, AGE 56 ———————————

IT'S NOT A SPRINT, IT'S A MARATHON

I became deeply invested in my clients' physical and emotional health, strength, and wellness, and I believed deeply in my ability to provide an outlet for them to achieve success. In our training sessions, I spent time getting to know my clients' physical histories, diets, and any injuries, as well as their fitness goals, in order to customize individualized programs. It didn't take long for my Pilates clients to see real changes.

People were coming to me with conditions such as osteoporosis, high blood pressure, obesity, and scoliosis. Imbalance, whether it's in the form of diet, muscle strength, or spinal health, can be the root of many problems. So my goal became, and still is, helping people balance their bodies.

For example, someone with scoliosis has a curvature in her spine that causes the back muscles on one side of the spine to be shorter and on the other side longer, while someone who carries extra weight in her abdomen tends to suffer back pain as the added weight begins to pull her spine forward. In both of these cases, spinal misalignment and muscular weaknesses can be improved by implementing Pilates movements to balance the front, back, and sides of the body.

Even those who are already in good condition will benefit from training their body in a balanced way. Imagine a runner who is very lean and has good muscle tone. The repetitive motion of running may cause the quadricep muscles in the front of the legs to be more dominant and stronger than the hamstrings on the back of the leg. Taking the time to do exercises that lengthen and strengthen the back of the leg and the hip flexors will not only balance the body but will improve the quality of the runner's stride and strength.

This holistic balancing of the body was another aspect of my personal training that made me stand out from day one. In fact, years later, after we opened Hilliard Studio Method, I received the kindest note from a marathon runner who had been suffering from hamstring injuries for more than a decade. After she started doing Hilliard Studio Method, she found that not only did her time improve, but she also stopped having issues with her hamstrings. It was incredible! She was so excited to find a method that exercised her full body and was core-centric, safe, efficient, results-oriented, and done in an hour.

s an ex-competitive collegiate runner and Olympic marathon trials qualifier, I have been plagued with chronic hamstring pain. Within a month of starting Hilliard Studio Method, I felt stronger and healthier running than I had in ten years, not to mention my "pre-two-kids" clothes fit better than ever! Additionally, the Method increased my flexibility in ways six years of yoga never did. I have done at least ten different barre-derived classes around the country during my work travels, and nothing comes even close to Hilliard Studio Method.

–FARRELL HUDZIK, AGE 40

In 2004, my family and I moved to a new home. We finally had enough space for me to set up my Pilates equipment and run my business from home! My clientele was growing right along with the space too, and I was honored to have some of Charlotte's top movers and shakers as clients. In fact, I was starting to have a bit of a wait list and began referring some clients out to other Pilates instructors whom I knew and respected.

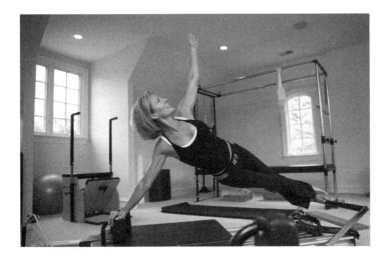

MAGIC IN THE MAKING

I was always creating and playing on my Pilates equipment in my free time, and I began to enhance various traditional movements into more customized workouts for my clients, based on their individual goals.

It didn't take me long to recognize that by incorporating non-traditional Pilates equipment, such as free weights, gliders, weighted balls, and stability balls, I could help my clients experience results they had not achieved in the past. I had a strong foundational knowledge from my classical Pilates training of anatomy and the importance of core strength and body control, but I believed I could find a more efficient and effective way to get immediate results. I was inspired by the challenge and excited about the prospect of developing a new method to transform client's bodies and minds in new ways.

The impetus that led me to find that missing piece came in 2007 when Clary, head over heels in love, told me she was getting married. We planned a wedding that would be a year away. Clary had one goal in mind: lean out and tone up. She wanted to transform her body, and she needed my help to do it. She was tall and beautiful, but she wanted more than what she was getting with her current routine. She'd been running five times a week and doing hot yoga two to three times a week. We attended quite a few yoga classes, where we were able to relax, laugh, and recite mantras together. All of those efforts produced a lot of sweat but not the physical changes Clary desired.

Creating the best possible exercise routine for Clary became my one and only mission. I began researching every exercise method I could find with the goal of crafting the most efficient and effective workout I could find not just for Clary but for me, too. At fifty-three years old, I was starting to see my body react more slowly to my traditional Pilates workouts.

I was an expert in Pilates and understood the importance of the core, but I wanted to see what other elements I could include to find that winning combination. I explored weight training, barre classes, yoga, martial arts, and athletic conditioning classes only to find that no single method worked the way I wanted. I never felt a perfect balance between cardio and strength training, balance and flexibility, the mental challenge and the emotional release. I was not going to be defeated by age or let my daughter down on her wedding, so I kept working and, in the process, discovered what's now known as Hilliard Studio Method.

Today, Hilliard Studio Method is shaping brides for their wedding days with our live classes and our bridal workout videos. No one works harder than a bride to get in shape for her wedding day; I learned that firsthand with Clary!

*J*ust wanted to say the biggest *thank-you* to everyone at the studio for helping me get into shape for my wedding! I honestly never thought I could be in this kind of shape for my big day, and to actually have toned arms for the first time in my life was a huge plus!

In the four months between buying my dress and my final fitting, I lost over five inches around my waist, went down to a size twenty-four in jeans, lost nine pounds, built abs, and gained strength everywhere. I never thought any type of workout in the galaxy could do anything like this to one person!

As a lifelong vegetarian, it's close to impossible for me to build strength and tone, but you proved me wrong again. I can look back on my wedding pictures, forever knowing how hard I worked to create a body I was confident in and extremely proud of! After all those "reach and squeezes," I never even noticed what it was doing to my back until I saw the pictures of me in my wedding dress!

Next stop: babies! So there will definitely not be any stopping at this point. Woohoo!

–NICOLA HEROY, AGE 32

TRANSFORMATIVE MOMENT

As Clary and I planned for her wedding, I took as many classes as I could all over the country, from Los Angeles to New York. Some were challenging and some were not, but in the process, we stumbled upon a new workout.

Barre classes were offered on both coasts, but they hadn't yet popped up in Charlotte. I knew that Lotte Berk, a German ballet dancer, had originally developed barre classes in the 1960s that focused on the core, spot training, and flexibility, but that was all I knew. Clary and I were shocked that people were paying up to forty dollars for these classes, but I could only assume it was worth it.

We absolutely loved the first barre class we took in New York City. We instantly felt the energy of the group class and could quickly feel the results of the small, intense movements.

It was one particular class that inspired me to look more closely at the way in which resistance training could enhance barre-based exercises. In that class, Clary and I experimented by picking up heavier weights than what the instructor suggested and what the other clients were using. The instructor went on to comment that Southern girls really liked to bulk up, but I knew I was onto something with the resistance as I felt my heart rate skyrocket and my muscles fatigue from using heavier weights.

THE FEAR OF BULKING

Weight lifting was an area I hadn't spent much time exploring, mainly because of the common myth that lifting weights would only make women bulk up. I wasn't going to leave a single stone unturned in my research, though, so I hired a hugely muscular and well-credited weightlifting personal trainer and said to him, "Your challenge is to bulk me up!"

He laughed and said, "I don't think I can bulk you up, but I'll give it a shot."

He tried, and for six solid weeks I worked out like a bodybuilder, lifting heavy weights. At the end of that time, I started to notice one change that I didn't expect at all: my waist was shrinking. I was sculpting my body and slimming down, not getting bigger and bulkier.

As a Pilates instructor focused on the core, I was shocked to see my waist suddenly getting smaller and my abs getting flatter, and I hadn't bulked up a bit. Why? Because most women have significantly less testosterone than men, which means it is very difficult for them to gain muscle the way men can. More importantly, I wasn't consuming the high-caloric diet needed to build my body. Not only did I have a smaller waist after six weeks but, for the first time, I had cut arms and, most surprisingly, this nice, new definition in my legs that had never been anything more than skinny. Everything about my shape was changing, and I loved it!

It was that time spent weight lifting that led to the real genesis of Hilliard Studio Method: the moment I realized the power of adding heavy resistance to core-centric work. This type of resistance, using weights up to ten pounds, sculpted, toned, and shaped my muscles more quickly, and I found I could also safely increase my heart rate to a healthy level without having to incorporate high-impact exercises.

In addition to traveling all over the country to explore different workouts, I spent hundreds of hours reading articles from leaders in the fitness industry. I wanted to know the real science behind all forms of exercise. I dug up research papers, scientific journals, numerous studies, and clinical trials. The physical benefits of exercise didn't surprise me, but I began to learn more about how the benefits of exercise can also positively impact your overall lifestyle, from what you eat to how you sleep. I kept this knowledge in the back of my mind about how important it was to create not just a physical exercise method but also a lifestyle based on holistic health. I've always said vanity goes a long way as inspiration, but the long-term effect of exercise on your physical and mental state is what matters the most.

> "I don't want to bulk up." Could this fear be keeping us from doing the exercises that will help us achieve the slim, toned body we dream of?

THE FEAR OF BULKING: A SCIENTIFIC AND PERSONAL EXPLORATION

"I don't want to bulk up." I hear it all the time. Could this fear be keeping us from doing the exercises that will help us achieve the slim, toned body we dream of?

Science proves higher resistance with fewer reps does not produce "bulk" and actually burns more calories and boosts metabolism more than lower resistance with higher reps. In a *New York Times* article, science writer Anahad O'Connor states that producing bulky muscles requires exceptionally high-calorie consumption, much over two thousand a day. He cites three studies, one in which one group of female subjects lifted weights at 85 percent of their ability, eight times, and the other group, 45 percent, fifteen times. The group of women lifting heavier weights burned more calories while performing the exercise and had higher metabolic rates than the group lifting lighter weights. [1]

---

1 Anahad O'Connor, "The Claim: For Better Muscle Tone, Go Lighter and Repeat," *The New York Times,* April 5, 2010, http://www.nytimes.com/2010/04/06/health/06real.html?_r=0.

HILLIARD STUDIO METHOD IS BORN

A few months before Clary's wedding, I finally had something that was a total-body workout combining all of my research into the ideal fitness program. Now all we needed to do was try it. Clary and Laura, one of my dear friends and clients, were my guinea pigs, and together we worked out four times a week in my private studio.

Every day, I would come in excited by the challenge of developing this new method, working us out, and pulling all of my ideas together into a cohesive routine. We would pick up our weights and see how all of the different combinations of moves I had created made our bodies feel.

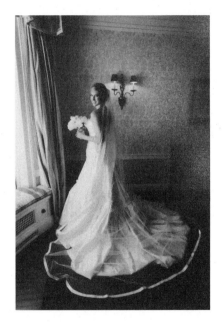

My goal was to create a workout that accomplished everything in one hour. I wanted to be a one-stop shop: sixty minutes of heart-pumping resistance and toning all done in a safe manner so that the workout could be done daily. I wanted something that I had never experienced before.

And it worked! We all started seeing changes, and Clary, who is six feet one inch tall, went from a size ten to a size four. It was stunning. *She* was stunning. I still remember when a friend told me, after seeing me walk down the aisle at Clary's wedding, "Whatever you all are doing in that studio, it works. I want to do it too because I want your back!"

With that, another lightbulb went off in my head. This workout I had created had changed Clary's body in her twenties, Laura's body in her thirties, and my body in my fifties. This workout was for every age and every body. I helped my daughter feel and look beautiful, and I knew I could deliver the same results to my clients of all different shapes, sizes, and ages. What started out with a single request from my daughter turned out to be the beginning of Hilliard Studio Method.

3
THE TAIL OF THE TIGER

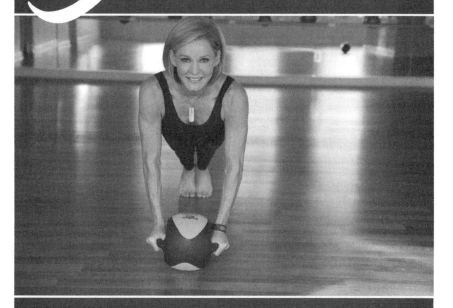

CHAPTER 3:
THE TAIL OF THE TIGER

After Clary's wedding, people called me left and right to tell me how great Clary and I looked, and my personal-training clients asked me if we could do what Clary and I had been doing. I started training small groups of clients in my home studio, using the five large pieces of Pilates equipment already packed in there, both for their intended purpose and as a barre, doing combinations of the new method with the Pilates reformer training.

My clients loved it, and one day someone said to me, "You need to open up a studio and charge forty-five dollars a person for this group class. You're going to kill it!" My mouth dropped open at her suggestion. I wasn't going to charge forty-five dollars per person, but I was willing to give this group class a try.

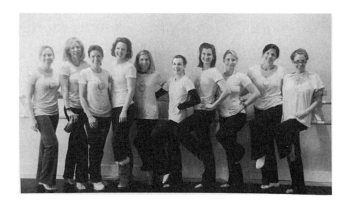

I found a local gym, the Cornwell Center, where I rented a space in the cycling room and taught three days a week, and through word of mouth, the number of clients at each class grew until the classes were full. I dealt with whatever equipment was in the room and integrated it into the workout however I could. That demand continued until I quickly outgrew the Cornwell Center and began looking for more space.

It didn't take long to find a local ballet studio that would sublease a classroom to me. It was just what I needed. I finally had a ballet barre! I started ordering equipment such as mats, bands, weights, and balls and was inspired to craft a new workout every time I saw a new piece of equipment.

A couple of weeks into the new studio space, I noticed that attendance was starting to drop, so to market my bare-bones business, I developed and e-mailed a weekly newsletter to remind clients I was there. Problem solved! Classes were filling, and I continued to send that weekly newsletter with my class schedule as well as health tips focused on fitness and nutrition and all aspects of health. These weekly emails reach our growing client list even to this day.

I am #54. What this means is a cool thing. It is like having a 212 area code when no more of them are given out. I started working out with Liz years ago, back when classes were taught a couple days a week at the Cornwell Center. My member number is, yes, that old.

Hilliard Studio Method was amazing from the start, as many of us know, and now years later, I still love the class and am a regular. All of the girls from those days back at the Cornwell Center are also still regulars.

There are two things that kept me coming back to class week after week:

1. I love working out and do it every day. I will try just about anything, and if I am in New York City or traveling anywhere else, I will try the best of what is available. This validates for me what Liz has developed. The Method is the most efficient workout I have tried anywhere. And Liz continues to keep it cutting edge. (My sister insists on taking classes when she is in town because she can't get this type of workout anywhere else.)

2. My life and my four wonderful children motivate me to work out, and I love to run. This kind of cardio is not the same as what I get at Hilliard Studio Method. The Method gives me an hour of cardio plus serious toning, and in class, I push myself much further than I would ever do on my own. I have become a better and stronger runner because of the work I do in class.

Oh—and I will list a third point: the best part of all is that Hilliard Studio Method is a lifestyle where I find not just a wonderful workout but food and health tips to keep my family and me healthy.

–AMY HINES ───────────────────────────────

CLARY'S "BE POWERFUL" MOMENT

Meanwhile, it wasn't long after Clary's wedding that she and her husband moved to Cambridge so he could attend Harvard Business School. She called me, concerned about the struggles of finding a job in a new town. A UNC-Chapel Hill graduate, she had worked in the marketing department of a prominent law firm in Charlotte. Since college she had defined herself as a "corporate woman," but something was shifting inside her. She missed the excitement and creativity we had together working out and preparing for her wedding.

"You know what?" she said to me over the phone. "I'm going to follow my passion, and I don't care if that doesn't sound as impressive as working for a PR agency or a corporate law firm because this is what I love to do."

Clary started practicing the Method in her five-hundred-square-foot apartment, using her husband's desk as a makeshift barre and coordinating the moves with music.

We were on the phone together every day, talking through the routines. I sent her some training videos, and she signed on to complete a national fitness instructor and barre-training program in Boston.

Clary's "Be Powerful" moment was in realizing how truly passionate she was about teaching our method and helping people feel better, inside and out. And what was even more amazing was that the Harvard community truly celebrated and supported her for following her passion and acting on her dreams.

The first class Clary taught was in the complex she lived in, a modern Harvard graduate student housing building with an atrium overlooking the Charles River. Of course, there wasn't a ballet barre there, but as we always do, she improvised, this time with a three-foot-tall wall that just happened to dissect the room. Her first class had only three people, but very soon word spread, and she began teaching sold-out classes several times a week at the student housing building and at Harvard's undergraduate, law school, and business school gyms.

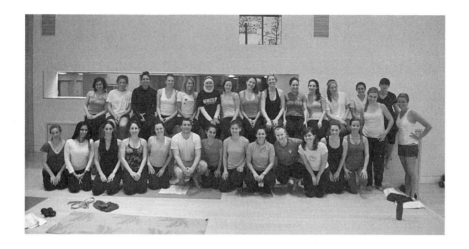

For a while, it tickled us to say that Hilliard Studio Method was a chain, with locations in Charlotte, North Carolina, and in Cambridge, Massachusetts. We even had T-shirts made with the two locations listed, which was funny, in a way, because only Clary and I were teaching classes, but it was also a moment of pride and realization: I realized that Hilliard Studio Method could exist on a much grander level than part-time classes in subleased spaces, and I began to set my sights on the future.

In the meantime, Clary's classes continued to grow, and I found myself constantly going back and forth on the phone with her, sending e-mails and, literally sometimes only an hour or so before a class, going over new moves and entire routines. She would pore over her notes in a much more organized fashion than I've ever done, and then she would teach an imaginary student in her room by herself and call me anytime she ran into a snag with the routine.

I'll never forget when she called me up after her first time subbing for a Pilates class at Hemenway Gym, the Harvard Law School gym. She didn't call it Hilliard Studio Method, but that was what she taught, and afterward, group attendees, including a few professors, ran up to her and said, "That's the best Pilates class I've ever been to!"

Well, hot damn, thought Clary, and I couldn't have said it better myself. We knew we had something, but for Clary to hear that kind of feedback after teaching her very first Pilates class was an incredible affirmation of her decision to teach!

FEELING LIKE ROCK STARS

It was around that time, when we started cheering about our "chain" of Hilliard Studio Method locations, that some of our clients began asking us about our business plan and if there might be any opportunities to invest in it.

We didn't really know what to tell them. *Invest in what?* we thought. There was nothing really to put money into since we didn't have worth yet or even a business plan—just a program.

Even without a business to invest in, the Harvard community continued to support Clary. And as graduation day for her husband rolled around in 2010, Clary saw that support in overwhelming abundance.

As a special treat for her husband's graduating class, Clary offered a Hilliard Studio Method class with me as the guest instructor. When I showed up to teach the class, I couldn't believe what I saw: the room was absolutely packed with men and women, and they treated me like a rock star.

The class we did that day was about as raw as you can get. We had nothing to work with, and even if we had, there wouldn't have been enough equipment to go around that huge crowd, so I drew on my strengths and improvised.

It was intense and fun, and the energy in that room was electric. There's just something about Clary and me getting together to teach a class; the intensity between us is tangible, and our class felt that.

They were going through every move with smiles on their faces, thriving on our energy.

In the midst of it all, I remember looking over at Clary, both of us with these huge grins on our faces, and she said to me, "Maybe we've got something here. This might actually work out."

I knew we could do this together and it would be amazing, so I replied, "So when are you coming home?"

THERE'S ONLY ONE LIZ AND CLARY

Clary decided to come home in the summer of 2010, not long after her husband graduated, and truly, she couldn't get back soon enough.

I was so pumped that, even when the landlord of the ballet studio I'd moved to started to take issue with me over some of the class times and rent, it didn't really faze me. My daughter was coming home, and we were going to blow this business out of the water.

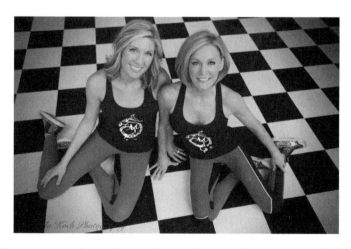

Then, one night, as I was driving home after a particularly rough rental discussion with the landlord, I happened to look up and, literally, just down the street, was a brand-new sign for Pure Barre, the largest, most successful barre studio chain in the United States. As I read the words on that sign, that old feeling of powerlessness swept over me as heavily as it had so many years ago, and I realized for the first time how important Hilliard Studio Method was to me. It wasn't just my business, it was my baby—and Pure Barre was going to kick my ass.

I had put my heart and soul into Hilliard Studio Method, and I knew what I had was great, but I also knew how established and successful this new competition was. Before that moment, I felt that I could walk away from my business if I needed to, but in that moment, as scary as it was, I knew I was going to stand up, work hard, trust my instincts, and protect and grow Hilliard Studio Method beyond anything Pure Barre or any other studio could ever touch.

They had every resource, every cool piece of equipment, and they knew what they were doing. And here I was, trying to make it all work, part time, out of a subleased ballet studio. I'd resolved to fight it out in the shadow of a barre-chain giant, but I had no idea how I was going to do it.

In the midst of that feeling of powerlessness, I was fortunate to receive the advice of my friend Laura, my client who was the Method's guinea pig and had been with me since the beginning. She had come over for our still-weekly personal training sessions, when I confided in her about my business fears. Laura had become a huge success on her own since those first Hilliard Studio Method days, opening a local, high-end women's clothing boutique.

When I told Laura about Pure Barre, she looked at me intently and said, "You feel exactly the way I felt when Neiman Marcus came to Charlotte. At the time, I was wondering how I could possibly compete with someone so big, just like you're wondering now how you can possibly compete with Pure Barre."

"But here's the thing," she said. "What they don't have is *you*. And what they *don't* have is your workout. Just keep doing what you do best. Keep giving that personal service and personal connection, and they won't be able to touch you."

It was an inspirational and empowering moment not just because she made me feel better about the situation and my workout but because it was the first time a client had seen my vulnerability. The empowering energy that I had always given my clients was now being given back to me.

> "What they don't have is *you*. And what they *don't* have is your workout.

I don't think Hilliard Studio Method even had a blip in attendance once Pure Barre opened. They were offering twelve classes a day between 5:30 a.m. and 9:00 p.m., and I could still only offer about three classes a week, but our attendance rates soared. This gave me the confidence and encouragement to keep my chin up, work hard, and do what I do best.

HSM BEYOND BARRE

I called my classes HSM Beyond Barre for a time because that's such an integral part of what Hilliard Studio Method is: it's not a static workout; it's evolutionary. From the very beginning, I evolved the Method past Pilates and then quickly evolved past barre too, never focusing on just one piece of equipment or one muscle group. We teach some classes in which we don't even need the barre.

Hilliard Studio Method is a powerful, nimble, all-encompassing program that is constantly changing, constantly surprising and invigorating the body, and constantly keeping our clients interested because it's never the same workout twice. At Hilliard Studio Method, we're original, we're creative, and we have the ability to help people change their bodies and their mind-sets in powerful ways. In changing my mind-set about the new studio next door, I knew that we were more than capable of being not just competitive with, but standing out above, any other workout.

FINDING OUR HOME

In 2013, we made a giant leap of faith and moved into a bigger studio that was all our own. Up to that point we'd been subletting, first from Cornwell and then from the ballet studio, but this place was ours entirely. And it was huge! I remember the first time we walked in. Clary looked around and said, "This is nice! It would be

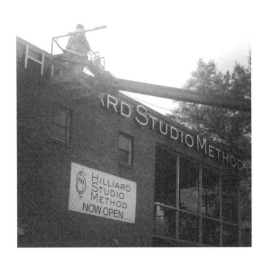

great in about five years." But I was hooked. I signed the lease without another thought and we moved into the space with record speed. During our first week that August, every one of our classes was free, and those who'd been with us since the Cornwell days got a letter, written and delivered by Clary and me, and a shirt that said "HSM for Life" as a thank-you for their support.

It's been amazing ever since. That move was when we truly took off as a business. Until then, we'd offered classes where we could, part time, working around other people's schedules, but now we literally ruled the roost!

When we opened the doors of our flagship studio with a skeleton staff, we had no idea if we'd have the clientele needed to support such a large space. We needed more classes, not only because of our rapidly growing client base but also because of all the overhead we were now responsible for: teaching staff, desk staff, and rent, along with advertising, lawyers, and other business costs. I felt I was holding the tail of a tiger. It was fast, furious, and not to be stopped. So what did we do? We took the only logical next step: we built a website, shot a workout video, and celebrated the launch of both with a party so fabulous that it made the next-day news!

We invited everyone we could think of, including all the stars and well-known names in Charlotte, as well as local media, and the next day, that party was all anyone could talk about. Meanwhile, we barely had enough money to pay for the caterer and had to put the videographer on a payment plan.

We still weren't making enough to pay ourselves, but we had enough to pay our bills and enough energy, support, drive, and determination to realize, once again, that we absolutely had something great here—and we were going to be a huge success not only for ourselves but also for our clients, who had so loyally supported us.

I stand in a long line of enthusiastic supporters for Liz, Clary, and all the trainers at Hilliard Studio Method. Just see the wonderful testimonials! During my commercial real estate years in Atlanta and throughout NC, plus travelling for fun, I have never worked with nor experienced a more contagious, challenging workout concept. Seeing Liz and Clary grow the Hilliard Studio Method "baby" over the years is witness to the success of the Method. This is a highly efficient hour packed with building strength and mental toughness. As a phenomenal by-product, inches melt. I kid you not. *Hilliard Studio Method changes your body.* Simultaneously, the brain is engaged with new positions, new props, new routines, and then the weight work and barre work might flip flop the next day, totally making more neuron connections.

Amazing how one's perspective changes over the years. At one hundred . . . okay, I'm fifty-five, but for our family, weight-bearing exercise is critical for skeletal health and joint issues. Our sweet mother suffered with osteoporosis and arthritis, and I refuse to be limited by genetics.

With Hilliard Studio Method, I know I can age gracefully with strength and power. I encourage any gal out there, no matter how young or old, to come and join in the fun.

Another benefit? I just pulled out all my winter clothes and many items are all too loose by two inches, and this after four years of doing the Method—you never plateau. Thank you Liz and Clary for literally changing how Charlotte gals are looking and feeling!

PS: My husband thanks you gals every day!

–MOLLY TULL, AGE 55 ————————————————

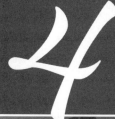

STRONGER THAN
TRAIN SMOKE

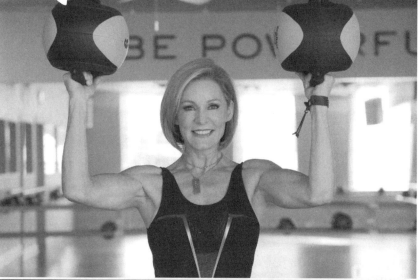

CHAPTER 4:

STRONGER THAN TRAIN SMOKE

Hilliard Studio Method is high energy, dynamic, constantly evolving and is a reflection of why we went into business in the first place: to help women change their bodies and develop physical, mental, and emotional strength. Clary and I stay energized knowing that we must evolve just as the workout does. We strive to bring our real, authentic selves to all that we do, and we know that the energy we bring to the table invigorates our diverse range of clients and makes us unstoppable!

WORK TO YOUR EDGE

Regardless of what we're teaching or the range of age in class any given day, we always say, "Work to your edge!" What is *your edge*? Your edge is the point where you wonder if you can do one more rep. When you push yourself to complete one more rep, you change your body and also your mind. And that's where you truly shine. We know the effort it takes to achieve success in our workouts, and we know that not everyone has the same edge. We care about our clients, taking the time to not only know them by name but also by their fitness levels and goals. We support their strengths and successes as well as their weaknesses and struggles, and cheer them on to their personal edge, nurturing and empowering them every step of the way. That's where our "Be Powerful" mantra comes into play again.

When I created this Method, it wasn't because I wanted to revolutionize the way we work out. I wanted to create the best, most efficient exercise for my daughter so she could be in the best shape of her life on her wedding day. But it did turn out to be a revolution in fitness. Hilliard Studio Method is the best of Pilates, barre, weight lifting, and yoga—the most efficient parts picked out and woven together into one beneficially muscle-confusing, spine-strengthening, total-body workout.

YOUR CORE CONNECTION IS ESSENTIAL

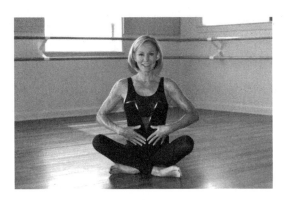

One of the most valuable things I have learned over the years about physical fitness is the power of core strength. The benefits of core strength include preventing injury, reducing and eliminating pain, balancing the body's muscle mass, and creating good posture.

Most people think their body's core is their belly or maybe their belly and a little bit of their back. But the truth is that your core is actually the area between your shoulders and hips. When we use the phrase *lock and load your core*, we mean that you should relax your shoulders down your back, open your chest wide, and pull your abdominal muscles in and "zip up" your rib cage as though you're putting on a tight jacket. This ensures that your muscles and spine are in proper form to begin the exercise.

At Hilliard Studio Method we teach core strength very deliberately, taking the time to walk clients through all the connections they need to make, from proper muscle engagement and spinal alignment to breathing. Finding your core connection begins with breathing.

Try inhaling through your nose and then deeply exhaling through your mouth. As you exhale, draw your belly button back to your spine. Then, as you inhale, bring your shoulders high up to your ears and exhale as you drop your shoulders down. We always start with and primarily focus on the deepest, most important abdominal muscle, the *transversus abdominus*. This powerhouse muscle is the foundation of your abdominals. It wraps around your body like a girdle from just below your belly button to your pelvic floor. The transversus abdominus lies just below your internal and external obliques and *rectus abdominus*, or six-pack muscle. Having a six-pack may look good, but you need a strong foundation to support it. A stronger *transversus abdominus* gives you not only a flat belly but a strong back. Connecting to the *transversus abdominus*, an incredibly important muscle no matter the exercise, allows a safer level of control so that you are less prone to injury.

Just as the *transversus abdominus* is the powerhouse muscle of the core, the spine is the literal backbone of your health. The strength and health of your spine is directly related to the strength and health of your entire body. As I was developing Hilliard Studio Method, I knew that working out with an engaged core and an aligned spine meant working out safely.

*A*s a chiropractic sports physician, I'm quite focused on the importance of posture and core strength to prevent back and neck pain. I emphasize to patients the importance of overall strength and conditioning and at the same time maintaining joint flexibility to prevent musculoskeletal injuries.

Hilliard Studio Method is an excellent strength and conditioning technique that addresses all of the above. I like to exercise and stay in good physical condition. I personally do Hilliard Studio Method and find it to be an amazing and challenging total-body workout. It really addresses the core, posture, and extremity tonicity.

Be persistent, and you will be very happy with the outcome both physically and mentally.

–JOHN J. PRIESTER, DC, AGE 62 ────────────

LOOK FIVE POUNDS LIGHTER

Want to immediately look five pounds lighter and gain an inch in height? Just stand up straight. Your posture can have a dramatic impact on your health and the way your body looks. Neck pain, back pain, and a belly pooch can be corrected and alleviated by improving your posture. So much of what we do in life—such as carrying a child, typing on a computer, driving a car, even trying to get warm on cold days—causes us to round the shoulders forward, creating shortened, tightened muscles in our shoulders and chest. Becoming self-aware is the first key to improving your posture. If you find yourself hunching, straighten up by pulling your shoulder blades together at your back—if you are a chronic huncher, you may feel you are sticking your chest out when you are actually in proper spinal alignment—then drop your shoulders down your back to make your neck long. Pull in your abdominal muscles for core support and a flattened tummy.

STRETCHES TO IMPROVE POSTURE AND OPEN UP THE CHEST

- **Weighted Foam Roller Stretch.** Place heavy weights (8, 6, or 5 lbs.) on either side of a foam roller. Lie vertically, head to tailbone, on the foam roller with your spine aligned down the middle. Keep your knees bent and feet flat on the floor with your belly button pulled down to your spine. Pick up the weights and bring them to your chest. Extend the weights straight up from your chest, palms facing. Inhale and slowly lower the weights down by the sides of your chest in a fly position, palms facing up. Don't let the weights drop lower than your shoulders. Exhale and slowly press the weights back together over your chest. Repeat ten times, making sure your back is gently pressed into the roller and your core is engaged throughout. If you have any type of shoulder injury, start with no weights and make a fist until you are comfortable using 3 lb. weights.

- **Doorway Stretch.** Stand in a doorway with one arm at ninety degrees, keeping your elbow level with your shoulder and hand directly above the elbow—what we call "field-goal" position. Then gently press your arm into the doorway structure and let your body lean forward as you feel the stretch across your chest. Repeat on your other side.

- **Clasped Hand Stretch.** Sitting or standing up straight, clasp hands together behind your back, pressing the heels of your hands together if possible, or hold on to the ends of a towel or strap. Lift your clasped hands up and away from your back and feel the stretch in your chest and shoulders.

THE SECRET OF THE SAUCE

I said earlier that the biggest secret to Hilliard Studio Method is that our routines are never the same twice. That may be the biggest secret to the structure, but the biggest secret to the sauce—to the actual rhythm of our fitness instruction—is that no matter what exercise we're doing, we're never focusing on just one muscle group. We don't just say, "Okay, today we're doing upper body," because we're not just doing upper body; rather, we're addressing the upper body, lower body, and core all at the same time. We focus on a primary muscle group while still engaging secondary muscle groups for a total body transformation.

That's the secret of the sauce.

It's simultaneous exercise that keeps the muscles confused and the heart rate up: a strategy that all trainers strive for and one that we feel we've perfected. We may do a bicep curl with a squat to kick off a class on Monday, but on Tuesday, we might pair your bicep exercise with a curtsy. Try balancing on your bare feet, while you hold your core in, keep your shoulders back and chest open as you complete a bicep curl. Those eight-pound weights are going to start feeling like twenty pounds, and your muscles are going to react as if they are too.

In every class, we ask you to listen to your body. Ask yourself if you can give more today. Some days will go more smoothly than others, so honor your body. Sore muscles are a sign of progress, but pain in the joints and neck are a sign of working out of alignment and out of position. The point of Hilliard Studio Method is to help you get stronger, sculpt a beautiful body, and sharpen your mind.

BURN CALORIES LIKE A 747 ON IDLE

I probably get more questions about cardio than anything else combined. First of all, running and cycling or doing any type of cardio is great for a strong, healthy heart, and you will burn calories while you're doing it. But minutes after your body cools, so does the calorie burn.

Unfortunately, the myth that cardio-only exercise is great for weight loss has been perpetuated far too long. The truth is cardio does little to increase your metabolism and can actually slow it down when done in excess because it decreases your muscle mass, which causes your body to burn fat at a slower rate.

Resistance training burns fat and calories at the highest rate possible while you work out, but even more importantly, while you're at rest. Hilliard Studio Method is designed to burn calories like a "747 jet on idle," making it stand out among other workouts. Our unique use of resistance training combined with fat-burning cardio improves both your cardiovascular endurance and your muscle tone.

Resistance Training at a Heart-Pumping Pace

+

Protein and Plant-Focused Eating

=

a Lean, Sculpted, Calorie-Burning Machine

BUT WON'T I BULK UP?

Many women who work out have a fear that if they train with too much resistance, they'll become bulky and big instead of sleek and slim. That's not what resistance training does. It doesn't bulk you up or out.

Resistance is key to building muscle, not bulking up muscle, because muscle building causes the body to burn more calories. In fact, muscles at rest burn five and a half times more calories than fat tissues (6.5 calories per pound, per hour with muscle compared to 1.2 calories per pound, per hour with fat).[2]

At the same time those muscles are burning those extra calories, they're also replacing adipose tissue, which is another word for that loose connective tissue we call fat. With resistance training, you're building muscle, and as it builds, it turns around and burns fat like crazy. Another plus? The kind of weight training we do at Hilliard Studio Method is an antiaging agent because it boosts your bone density too, helping to ward off or fight common bone diseases such as osteoporosis or osteopenia.

What's more, as I noted when I worked with a weight-lifting personal trainer, resistance training can reduce the size of the waist without having to run laps or pound the pavement. Most people, when they want to burn fat, think *cardio, cardio, cardio,* and start running. Instead, they should be thinking *resistance, resistance, resistance.*

I'm not telling you not to run, of course! Running is wonderful, and we have several marathoners who come to class regularly. But what you have to be careful of is burning through the calories and carbohydrates in your body and burning straight into your protein and muscle stores so that you're actually burning muscle away, losing it instead of strengthening it.

---

2   Nick NG, "How Many Calories Does a Pound of Muscle Burn Per Day?" Livestrong, February 4, 2014, http://www.livestrong.com/article/310070-how-many-calories-does-a-pound-of-muscle-burn-per-day/.

At the same time, your body is quick to adapt to long "same-speed" cardio workouts, reducing the number of calories you burn each time. And if you're doing it a lot, your metabolism no longer has that calorie-burning, lean muscle mass to work with. This is why we recommend weight training when you're trying to lose inches and sculpt your body, as it improves muscle tone, increases strength, and promotes metabolic health and fat loss.

So if you're running, don't stop! But *do* start working core-centric resistance training into your workout to keep those muscles strong and to prevent those all-too-common knee injuries. There you will find the magic potion for that killer body you've dreamed of!

EXERCISES YOU CAN DO AT HOME

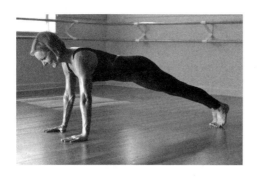

Plank: If you do anything today, hold a plank! It is one of the most efficient moves for your entire body. You may think you won't get your heart rate up, but try holding this position up to thirty, sixty, and even ninety seconds. Place your hands on the ground under your shoulders and extend your legs and push through the heels of your bare feet. You should be in a long line from your shoulders to your hips to your heels. Pull your belly button up toward your spine as you extend through the crown of your head to the base of your tailbone, never letting your shoulders creep up to your ears or your back round or arch. To make this easier, bend your knees and place them on the floor for a modified plank. To make this more difficult, try some single-leg lifts and side planks.

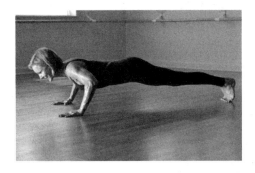

Push-ups: You can do these on your knees or, traditionally, with straight legs. Either way, you will be firing into your core and upper body. We do traditional wide-arm push-ups at Hilliard Studio Method to work into the chest, so make sure your hands are wider than your shoulders. Bend at the elbows and slowly lower your chest to elbow depth (not lower), and then press back up as you exhale and tighten your core. Try to complete ten at a time, adding more repetitions the stronger you get.

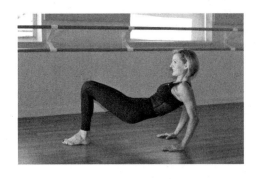

Triceps dancing: This move is perfect for preventing that dreaded under arm jiggle. Sit on your tailbone with your knees bent, and place your hands on the floor behind you under your shoulders. Keep your fingertips pointing toward your toes. Keep your core connected and strong as you lift and keep your hips off the floor. Bend your elbows until you feel the work in the back of your arms. Drive through the palms to return to straight. Make your goal forty dips even if you break between sets.

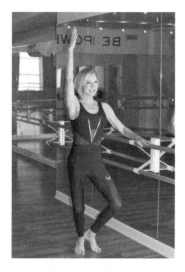

Narrow V: This is an excellent barre-based move for toning your thighs. Standing upright, place your hand on a table, chair, or wall. If you are already a pro at balance, raise both arms overhead like a ballerina. Place your heels together and don't let them come apart. Then open your toes four to six inches. Lift your heels off the floor one to two inches; imagine the shoe height of a "kitten heel." Bend your knees until your legs create a diamond shape and begin to move down one inch and then back up an inch. Alternate ten reps of this with ten reps of a faster one-inch pulse down. Hold nice and low for at least twenty seconds, and then repeat your set and get ready to see some good shaking.

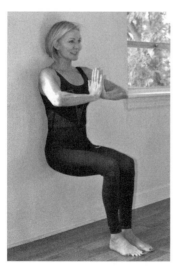

Chair: We do this move in class by pulling away from a barre, but you can get the same great results by sitting against a wall as you may have done in middle-school gym class! Lean your back against a stable wall and begin to slide down the wall until your knees are bent ninety degrees and directly in line over your ankles. Once you feel you are sitting in an invisible chair, you can hold stillness or add some challenging flair by lifting one leg off the floor, extending it, and holding for ten seconds.

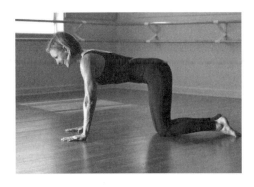

Tabletop: A go-to glute exercise, this tush toner is great for all levels. On all fours with your hands under your shoulders and your knees under your hips, pull in your belly and flatten your back. Lift one leg until it is parallel to the floor. Slowly begin to move your leg up one inch and down one inch by squeezing tightly with your glutes. Repeat twenty times. Next, bend your knee, bringing your heel to your seat. This will increase the work in the hamstring. Lift the bent leg up one inch and down one inch twenty times. Repeat the same moves on the opposite leg. Increase the work by placing the hand opposite your working leg on the small of your back to challenge your balance.

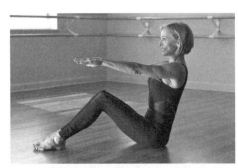

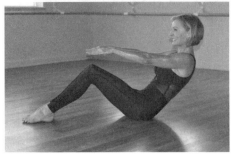

Abdominal roll downs and curl: Start in a seated position with your knees bent and your feet flat on the floor. Hold on to the backs of your thighs but keep your chest open. Tuck your tailbone under and scoop your belly button away from your shirt. Begin to slowly roll down one vertebra at a time while you

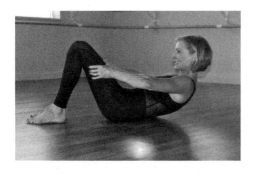

count to eight or ten until your head and shoulders are entirely on the ground. You will release your hands the lower you go but keep your feet grounded. Take a deep breath and pull your core in tight as your roll back up to the same seated position. This is both an excellent way to increase spinal flexibility and gain core strength. Complete several roll downs, and on your final one, stop halfway until your shoulders hover off the floor. This is a difficult position to hold, so if you are struggling, you will just hold a higher position until you can gradually roll down to a hover. In this curl position, hold your thighs, and keep your chin to your chest and your gaze straight ahead at your thighs. Your middle should be scooped out and pulled in and your shoulders relaxed. From here, gently curl up and over your stomach and then back down an inch. Hold at the top and gently pulse up an inch. Repeat as many curls as you can, and then hold the curl for thirty seconds. There's nothing better than feeling your abs work!

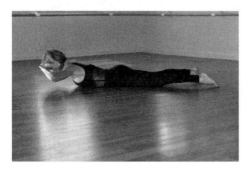

Back extensions: Lie flat on your stomach on the floor. Stack your hands and rest your forehead on them. Even though your stomach is on the floor, engage your belly button and try to pull it off the floor as much as you can. Gently lift one leg off the floor and then the other. As long as your low back feels good, try lifting both legs off the floor at once. When you get your thighs off the mat, gently squeeze through your glutes and low back and start to pulse up one inch. Rest as needed and repeat up to twenty lifts. Now bend your knees, lock your heels together, and flex your feet, imagining frog legs. Drive your heels to the ceiling and when your thighs are off the mat, begin to pulse up again twenty times. Advance this by lifting your arms, head, and chest off the floor, and pulse the lower and upper body up together. This important move keeps you balanced and strengthens both sides of your body.

Since high school, my fitness identity could pretty singularly be wrapped up as "runner." And as said runner, the only exercise I consistently made time for was…you guessed it…running. Sure, I enjoyed other things—hiking, yoga, etc. But those were just icing on the cake. The cake was always running. Eventually though (you see where this is going don't you?)…I did learn that yes, it turns out you can have *too much* cake. And as a pattern of nagging overuse injuries, especially in my knees, and muscle imbalances began to emerge in my body, I begrudgingly started incorporating weight training and core work to keep those at bay.

I am a primary-care physician and spend a fair bit of time counseling people at their annual exams about the contributions of diet and exercise to their overall health. When posing the question "What is your current exercise routine?", I started taking note that a very *large* percentage of my patients were answering that Hilliard Studio Method was an integral part of their routine. This was usually followed by "You *have* to try it," "It's *so hard*," and "You'll *love* it." After hearing this multiple times a day for over a year and actually passing the studio on my way to work, I decided enough signs were pointing in the direction that yes, indeed, I did have to try it.

I thought a good place to start was a DVD. The first time I did a Hilliard DVD in my living room, I was grateful to hear Liz and Clary explain that, yes, your legs should be shaking. Because not only was I shaking, but I was humbled, and I was hooked. I loved this new challenge and immediately felt this was a routine I could be passionate about!

Within a couple weeks, I started attending live classes and fell in love with the energy of the studio. It's hard to believe almost seven months have passed since my first class. I have loved seeing and feeling my body, and thankfully my knees, get stronger with each passing week and pushing myself to a new edge on a regular basis. I can't thank Hilliard Studio Method enough for their ongoing encouragement for me, and so many women all over Charlotte, to "Be Powerful."

–DR. MEREDITH FAULKNER, AGE 34 ————————

WHY I DON'T USE A SCALE

The waistline is the measurement of your health, and this is why I rely on my waist circumference and the way my clothing fits rather than on the number on the scale. When I was in my thirties, I was a clothing size eight, and I weighed about the same then as I do know. However, the difference is that my body is now composed of lean muscle rather than fat. At a healthy height weight ratio of five feet nine inches tall and 130–135 pounds, I now wear a size four instead of an eight. While I don't want to put too much emphasis on the exact numbers, I *do* want to ease your mind about the fact that you may initially see the number on the scale increase when you incorporate resistance training, as we do at Hilliard Studio Method, because your muscle weighs more than fat, but it takes up less space than fat. Eventually you will see the muscle you build burn up the excess fat, and your jeans will start to fall off your hips.

Prior to finding the gem that is Hilliard Studio Method, my workout routine consisted of spending days at the gym on cardio machines and lifting weights. I would take hot yoga classes when I could, but I was bored and mostly trying to maintain my weight. In fact, I weighed myself every day and placed an unnecessary value on the number on the scale. By combining cardio work and strength training in one workout at Hilliard Studio Method, my body got exactly what it needed in a much quicker time. Specifically, my core strength increased immediately. After just three classes, I experienced the "zipping-up" effect in my

> That number on the scale will never compare to having a strong and fit mind and body.

torso and was much more aware of my posture. My waist and lower body have tapered, and my upper body has never been so toned. That number on the scale will never compare to having a strong and fit mind and body."

–LEE KENNELLY, HILLIARD STUDIO METHOD DIRECTOR OF TRAINING, AGE 37

NO SHOES, NO SOCKS, NO NONSENSE

Our feet contain an astounding 25 percent of the body's bones, and each one of them has an important function. Encasing our feet in shoes and constantly walking on artificial surfaces weakens our feet by depriving them of the natural workout that the muscles require, eventually causing strength and fine motor skill losses that are vital for our feet to properly support our bodies. Instead, we call on the muscles of the ankle to take the load, which leads to further weakening of the foot muscles. There are all sorts of domino effects that can come from weak feet, including ankle and knee problems and even hip problems.

This is one of the reasons Hilliard Studio Method workouts are in bare feet. Standing in wide second position on the balls of your bare feet—or as we like to call it, "wearing those Saturday-night high heels"—is much tougher than doing it with big padded shoes on and much healthier not only for your feet but also for the balance of your entire body. At Hilliard Studio Method, we take the body as a whole and set the bar high to strengthen your body, literally from your head to your toes!

WEIGHT TRAINING THE HILLIARD STUDIO METHOD WAY

At some point, you've likely heard about the rotator cuff in your shoulder, probably not in the sense that you've heard people raving about how strong theirs is but more in the sense that you've met someone who has torn it and gone through a grueling recovery and possibly surgery. Just like all of the elements that make up Hilliard Studio Method, I don't take for granted the way we do weight training. You shouldn't press heavy weights overhead if you're not in good form and—yes, you guessed it—if you're not connected to your core and in proper spinal alignment. Unlike traditional weight lifting, which works large muscle groups first from the outside in, I've developed exercises that work from the inside out. In essence, the goal is to strengthen the small, connective muscles around your joints before strengthening the primary, larger muscle groups.

In any of our classes, you will consistently hear our instructors reminding you to drop your shoulders away from your ears and pull your abs in. When I see you're out of form and your shoulders are hunched over in one of our classes, I'm going to make darn sure that I fix your form before you complete another rep. When we train the body in proper alignment, we build bodies in proper alignment. So not only are you sculpting beautiful "coconut muscles"—as we like to refer to the deltoid, or shoulder, muscles—but you are also strengthening your supporting muscle groups, such as the four smaller muscles of the rotator cuff. As I like to say, "Vanity goes a long way in getting us to work out, but safety is king, ensuring that you can work out daily for as long as you live!"

First, I would like to thank Hilliard Studio Method for getting me in the best shape of my life. My struggle to find an effective, fun, and dynamic workout started at a very young age. When I was just fourteen years old, I was diagnosed with a rare form of leukemia called undifferentiated leukemia. I went through three and a half years of intense chemotherapy, which took its toll on my body. As a result, I am a cancer survivor, but I now have avascular necrosis (AVN). AVN is a joint disease where there is an interruption of blood supply to the bone, the bone tissue dies, and the bone collapses. I have AVN in both shoulders, both hips, both knees, and my left elbow.

Starting at fourteen years old, I couldn't just go for a run anymore. Some days, just walking hurt. I have had over ten orthopedic surgeries to care for my joints, including a total shoulder and total hip replacement, all before my thirtieth birthday. I also have had three children. Needless to say, finding an intense workout for my entire body was not easy to find. Thank goodness for Hilliard Studio Method! The great thing about the Method is that I can modify any exercise and still get the workout I crave and the results I want. Even when I am having a "bad joint day" or when I am nine months pregnant, I can go to class and know I did something great for my body.

My doctors are so impressed with my strength, flexibility, joint range of motion, and overall quality of life. I know everyone needs to exercise to stay healthy, but exercise is so much more to me. Hilliard Studio Method keeps my body healthy, stabilizes my joints, and actually decreases my joint pain. I have young children for whom I have to be strong and a hubby I want to look hot for. As long as I have Hilliard Studio Method, I know I can do both!

–MICHELLE NEUN, AGE 35 ─────────────────────

STRONGER *AND* SMARTER

If having a strong, healthy body isn't enough to get you out of your seat, then consider how exercise affects your cognitive ability by raising your IQ, warding off Alzheimer's disease and dementia, preventing and treating depression, and slowing the effects of aging!

Dr. John Ratey, a Harvard Medical School psychiatrist, ascertains that exercise is overwhelmingly beneficial for the brain, improving memory, focus, cognitive functioning, and mood, while the physical changes we see are more of a side effect.[3] In his book, *Spark*, Dr. Ratey writes that exercise improves our ability to learn and actually makes us smarter, even as we age, by increasing blood flow to the brain, creating a surge in protective neurochemicals and allowing the brain to grow.

The effects of physical exercise on the brain are dramatically more beneficial than memory exercises such as sudoku and crossword puzzles that doctors have prescribed in the past. Newest research illustrates that women who regularly engage in moderate exercise have a 50 percent decreased risk of dementia, and men and women who already have dementia or Alzheimer's have higher cognitive function-

---

3   "Worldwide studies and science support exercise for relieving symptoms related to ADD, OCD, anxiety, depression, addiction and aging," Sparking Life, http://sparkinglife.org/page/why-exercise-works.

ing when they exercise than those who are sedentary.[4] Dr. Ratey's equation for brain health looks like this:

Keeping Your Weight Down

+

Exercise for the Brain + Body*

=

Healthy Brain
*(by far the most robust factor in the equation)

Studies also indicate the positive effects that exercise has on mood, hormonal changes in women, and overall state of happiness. One study Dr. Ratey referenced even showed that a brisk, twenty-minute walk a day is just as effective for treating mild depression as taking Zoloft.

The body is built and designed for the brain to survive and recreate itself through physical activity. If you stop moving, your brain begins to deteriorate. Most people work out because it's good for their body, but research continues to prove that the brain depends on exercise not only to survive but also to thrive. The side effect of exercise is a smokin' hot body.

---

4   "Brain cells and their connections degenerate as we age; aerobic exercise sparks new growth to optimize brain function," Sparking Life, http://sparkinglife.org/page/aging.

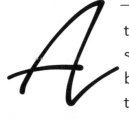

t twenty-five, I've experienced my fair share of health issues—from traumatic brain injury and a celiac disease diagnosis to respiratory inflammation and chronic fatigue. These unrelenting issues interrupted the quality of my life so severely that I left college after my junior year. Since then my health and quality of life has improved, but I felt like something was still missing. I started taking Hilliard Studio Method Essentials twice a week. In three short months, my body has changed inside and out! I have better posture, am lean and toned, but I've noticed other changes. I am less fatigued and more alert. Sticking to an exercise regimen requires discipline and focus, and that has been translated to other parts of my life. I have also seen a reduction of my pesky symptoms from celiac. Liz has developed an amazing method. The mental and physical healing value of exercise that I get at Hilliard Studio Method is worth every penny. I love the Method so much that I've asked for a year of classes for my college graduation this spring!

–HANNAH TRAVIS, AGE 27

FROM PREGNANCY TO POST-MENOPAUSE: HILLIARD STUDIO METHOD AT ANY AGE

One of our favorite sayings at Hilliard Studio Method is not only "Be Powerful" but "Be Powerful at any age" because you can be. Whether you're a bride-to-be or a retiree, you can tap into your strength and look and feel beautiful from the inside out.

At sixty-two years old, I am teaching and taking my workout almost daily. People approach me to discuss how exercise is antiaging, which it is! Working out to feel healthy and strong is imperative, and our clients who range in age from seventeen to seventy-one (*yes, seventy-one!*) years old have seen big-time benefits from the workout, not only becoming physically stronger, more flexible and toned, but also more mentally and emotionally adept.

HILLIARD STUDIO METHOD AND PREGNANCY

I was beyond thrilled when Clary announced in 2011 she was expecting her first baby—my baby was having a baby! Clary both taught and took Hilliard Studio Method classes regularly throughout both of her pregnancies, to which she credits her elevated energy level and pain-free pregnancies, healthy deliveries, and quick recoveries postnatal.

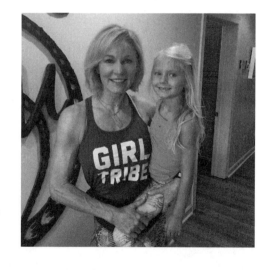

We filmed *Powerful Pregnancy*, a thirty-five-minute total-body workout that is a must for every mother-to-be, when Clary was seven months pregnant with her second child. But to turn around sixteen weeks postnatal and film *Total Body Workout* is the true testament to the effectiveness of our workout when bouncing back after baby!

About 10 percent of our clients are pregnant at any given time. They continue to come to class because they know our workout is effective and safe during pregnancy, but also because it makes them feel and look their best in a time that can be uncomfortable and bring out insecurities about body image. We often joke that the studio could be mistaken for a maternity ward, but I'll tell you, we have the strongest, healthiest mamas-to-be in the country.

Through extensive research and experience with countless clients and our own trainers, we have perfected modifications to our workout specifically for pregnancy. Our goal is to help women become strong and healthy so they can get pregnant, to keep them feeling good and their babies healthy throughout pregnancy, and to support them as new mothers when baby arrives.

Take the story one of our moms told us about the most amazing compliment she'd ever received. Before she came to Hilliard Studio Method, one of our clients named Hope had struggled with Crohn's disease and had never been able to workout consistently. But once she started, she was all in, standing in the first row four times a week.

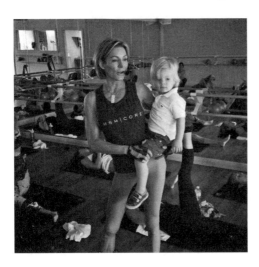

At eight months pregnant, she was attending a cocktail party when a female TV anchor came up to her and said, "Please don't take this the wrong way, but you have the nicest ass of anyone I've ever seen." "Wow," Hope said with a huge grin, "You just made my week!"

Another client, Tara, told us that she was able to fit in her pre-pregnancy jeans just three weeks after giving birth. *Three weeks!* That's not only impressive; it's inspiring.

Regular, safe exercise is not only great for helping mom maintain her strength, but it's also incredibly beneficial to the baby. Regular exercise during pregnancy boosts brain development in babies, according to a study presented at the Society for Neuroscience's annual meeting.[5] While researchers hypothesize on exactly why, this latest study of human newborns and their mothers shows that even moderate exercise three times a week causes their brains to be more mature than the brains of newborns of sedentary moms.

So that's why between our brain-boosting workout and healthy Hilliard Studio Method lifestyle, we say we're growing super babies at Hilliard Studio Method!

*P*ersonally, I credit Hilliard Studio Method with helping me get my body and body image back into a healthy state post surgery woes related to my Crohn's disease. Many people do not know that I have a seven-inch vertical scar on my stomach. However, thanks to Hilliard Studio Method, I rocked a bikini for the first time in over two years on an anniversary trip last May! I truly believe that the Method has played a *big* part in my journey to remission with Crohn's disease—I would not have been

---

5   Gretchen Reynolds, "Mother's Exercise May Boost Baby's Brain," *The New York Times,* November 20, 2013, http://well.blogs.nytimes.com/2013/11/20/mothers-exercise-may-boost-babys-brain/?smid=tw-share&_r=3&.

able to safely conceive and carry a baby if my body was not in remission. She is our biggest blessing!

Now, having become a mommy, more than ever I want to set a good example for my little girl. Hilliard Studio Method will be that slice of "me time," but it will also show my daughter the importance of taking care of herself and being healthy. During this stage in my life, the Method helped me feel strong and fit despite my growing waistline. I feel confident in my strength and in my ability to bounce back postpartum. Thankfully, I had a quick and easy delivery, much of which I attribute to Hilliard Studio Method. I truly felt strong and powerful.

For all women who have not tried Hilliard Studio Method, all I can say is, do not be intimidated! There are women of all different ages, shapes, and sizes, and all in different levels of their own personal health journeys in every class. From the second you walk into the studio, you're greeted with a smile and an awesome "girl power" vibe . . . it's such a welcoming atmosphere. I am so thankful for my Hilliard Studio Method family and am so happy to have a little HSMer in the making in my sweet, little Evie!

–HOPE SKOURAS, AGE 26 ——————————————

HILLIARD STUDIO METHOD'S APPROACH
TO WORKING OUT PREGNANT

The first trimester starts with three golden rules: tell your trainer so she can discreetly begin giving you modifications, hydrate more than usual, and take breaks as often as you need. During this time you probably notice you get winded after a simple walk up the stairs and start to sweat as soon as you begin moving, maybe even feeling light-headed. Follow these golden rules and know that you will feel more like yourself in the second trimester.

Once you enter the second and third trimesters, Hilliard Studio Method's experienced trainers will continue to provide modifications appropriate to your stage of pregnancy.

For example, in lieu of twisting and intense abdominal exercises you will hold a high plank and pike often, stretching out the tightened back body caused by your growing baby pulling your body forward. The abdominal-intensive section of class is replaced by additional arm and gluteal work, improving strength that will be needed throughout pregnancy, in delivery, and most importantly, for the snuggles soon to come!

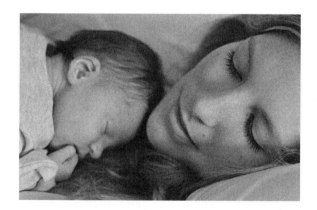

When I found out that I was pregnant, I was over the moon. But, like most women, a lot of worries accompanied that excitement. For one, I was worried about my figure and what the recommended twenty-five to thirty-five pounds of baby weight would do to it. My doctor encouraged me to exercise as much as I had prepregnancy, so I continued with my current workout regimen. At the time, that included about two days a week of Hilliard Studio Method plus spinning and other Pilates workouts.

I kept up that cocktail of workouts until I was a week or two into the second trimester. I started informing all of my exercise instructors before class that I was pregnant, but the Hilliard Studio Method instructors were the only ones to ever offer any modifications or suggestions for how to make my workout both safe and effective. Hilliard Studio Method is a challenging workout but is "pregnancy-friendly," as the instructors constantly cue modifications for anyone that is pregnant or that has an injury. The rest of my workout instructors just advised me to do what I "felt comfortable doing." Unfortunately, that didn't really help me. I felt "comfortable" doing almost everything, but I was worried I was going to hurt myself or my baby. I decided I was done with the other workouts and was going to stick to the Method 100 percent.

After a few weeks of going to Hilliard Studio Method four to five days a week, Clary stopped me after class one day and told me that she thought I was more toned than I was prepregnancy. I couldn't believe it, but when I looked at myself in the mirror, I had to agree she was right! I've consistently gone to Hilliard Studio Method since then, and I am impressed with the marked definition in my arms and thighs. Everyone warned me about pregnancy cellulite, but I can honestly say I have not seen any! Furthermore, I have not had any back pain, which I attribute to the plank series along with the back and shoulder work we do. Also, each day that I am in the studio, at least one Hilliard Studio Method instructor or staff member asks me how I am feeling or about my pregnancy.

As I've entered the last few weeks of pregnancy, I've certainly slowed down a bit, but I still keep at it. Hopefully all of these weeks of plank holds and pretzels will help me in labor and delivery and, most importantly, getting my prepregnancy body back!

–MEGHAN LLUBERAS, AGE 32 ————————

HOT-FLASH HOTTIE

I was lucky. I developed this Method at the same time I was going through menopause. Clary was getting married and her twenty-year-old body was reacting quickly to the workout. I was shocked that despite the hormonal changes I was experiencing that I was still able to see positive results. I was astounded that my waistline could shrink and my muscles could tone as I approached my midfifties. Clary and I were both getting in the best shape of our lives, and although I was already in great shape as a Pilates personal trainer who made working out and eating well a priority in my life, the additional physical benefits of my workout made the biggest difference. The Method was evolving and so were our bodies, and the results were undeniable.

What this Method delivers is a strong, sculpted body at any age. It helps you gain bone density and balance your hormones through its emphasis on resistance training, but not just any resistance training.

I asked one of our clients who is a primary-care physician to help me support this philosophy by sharing her thoughts about a medical journal article I had read, and here's what she had to say.

*W*omen often come into my primary-care office complaining, "Things just aren't like they used to be in terms of my metabolism. I am eating the same things, and doing the same amount of exercise, and still my weight is creeping up!"

The Surgeon General, in *Healthy People 2010*, recommends 150 minutes of moderate exercise per week (thirty minutes, five days a week), but is this really enough? Finally, there is some good medical literature that sheds some light on this subject. In an article published in JAMA (Journal of the American Medical Association), March 2010, a group from Harvard Medical School shared their findings of a large clinical trial in which they followed over thirty-four thousand premenopausal women for fifteen years and charted their weight and activity level while allowing them to consume their "usual healthy diet." Two key points are worth noting:

1. Just to *maintain* their weight, these women needed to exercise an average of sixty minutes per day *every day*. Yikes!

2. Only the women of normal weight (BMI less than twenty-five) were able to maintain their weight at all… subjects who approached menopause either over-

weight or obese tended to continue gaining weight despite their efforts at diet and exercise.

At first glance, this data might seem frustrating or even demoralizing (or *motivating* for some of us). What is clear, however, is that premenopausal women should strive to reach a goal of normal weight (BMI of 18.5-25) by the time of expected menopause if they are to have a fighting chance of maintaining their healthy weight (and lean physique) going forward. Many women in this age category need to ramp up their activity to the recommended amount of sixty minutes a day so that they can continue to feel and look their best not just today but for years to come. Remember, health first, aesthetics second!

Thank goodness Hilliard Studio Method offers us sixty action-packed minutes, seven days a week to enjoy the journey of continued fitness together!

–DR. ANNE BARNARD SCHMIT, AGE 47 ——

So what this tells us is that a safer yet more challenging workout on a consistent basis is the key to helping us physically age more gracefully. A study published by *Medicine & Science in Sports & Exercise* found that almost any amount and type of physical activity may slow aging deep within our cells.[6]

---

6   Gretchen Reynolds, "Does Exercise Slow the Aging Process?", *The New York Times,* October 28, 2015, http://mobile.nytimes. com/blogs/well/2015/10/28/does-exercise-slow-the-aging-process/?smprod=nytcore-ipad&smid=nytcore-ipad-share&_r=0&referer.

Being physically fit is a natural part of who I am and, I feel, is a natural part of everyone. We may not always feel we have the resources, time, or energy to work out, but when we do make that a priority, we are giving ourselves the greatest gift. Working out has gotten short shrift in our society as something self-indulgent, but it is a necessary part of health. The impact of exercise doesn't just improve how you feel but can also help you sleep better, reduce your risk of heart disease, and improve your bone density—all issues that women find themselves dealing with more and more as they age. You don't just have to read a study to know that after you work out, and sometimes during, you feel so much better than you did beforehand.

*E*very woman wants to look and feel her best, and Hilliard Studio Method meets all those needs. Besides the outward physical benefits, perhaps the most important things of all are the benefits that aren't so visible: increased flexibility, core strength, better mind/body connection, and most of all, better bone strength. I have the typical body type to have osteoporosis at my age, but thanks to the Method, my bone density is excellent.

Almost a year ago, I walked into Hilliard Studio Method, both excited and more than a little bit intimidated. I had known of Hilliard Studio Method for quite a while and had been thinking of giving it a try for several months.

I had exercised regularly all my life—various classes (who remembers step class?!), yoga, Pilates, running then walking, and strength work with a trainer. Though all of them were helpful in their own way, I felt I had hit a plateau and was ready to be pushed a bit more. After the first class, I definitely realized there was a whole other level of being in shape!

From the beginning, the entire Hilliard Studio Method team made me feel welcome, stressing to always listen to my own body. I learned it is okay to modify when my bad knees just don't allow me to do deep bends, and to drop to a lower weight when I feel I have reached my edge. The encouraging, positive, and friendly attitude of all the trainers and staff makes me feel comfortable even though most of the HSMers are young enough to be my daughter.

I am so grateful to Liz, Clary, and all the amazing trainers for making it possible to "Be Powerful" at any age!

–CAROLYN KILLINGSWORTH, AGE 71 ⸻

Hilliard Studio Method goes far beyond just making you look and feel your best. At every age and every stage, women are raving about the results that keep them healthy and coming back for more. We strive for efficiency and safety in the workout, and it delivers results. A fit lifestyle, however, doesn't stop with regular exercise. It also depends on a healthy and well-balanced diet. What you put into your body is an essential part of a healthy lifestyle, and when you eat well, you feel better about yourself. That, combined with a well-balanced exercise routine, can keep you feeling stronger than train smoke!

5
HILLIARD STUDIO
METHOD JET FUEL

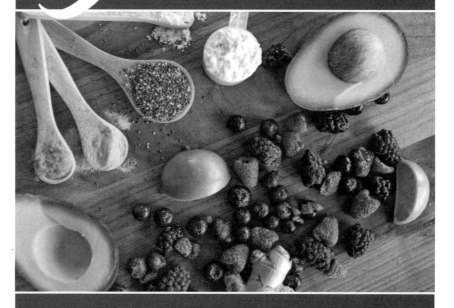

CHAPTER 5:
HILLIARD STUDIO METHOD JET FUEL

Healthy eating has always been an important part of life for Clary and me. No one's perfect, and I've caught myself with a handful of Raisinets at the movie theater on occasion, but our general *mode de vie* is to eat a healthy, well-balanced diet of real foods.

But what does that mean? It seemed like a simple answer to me: just eat what grows from the earth and forget the chemicals and added sugar. But early on, I found that a lot of people truly weren't aware of how harmful so much of the food out there can be.

Before we moved into our present-day studio, and even before the ballet studio, I remember teaching a class in our Cornwell Center space. The room was packed, the music was jamming, and while the group could hear me over all of that, it wasn't particularly easy to hold a conversation.

But right in the middle of class, one of my clients yelled out, "So what's the problem with high fructose corn syrup in your diet? Why can't I have that?"

I literally stopped dead in my tracks. The question had come from the wife of a prominent doctor in Charlotte, so I was a little surprised at first that she didn't know more about it. But the more I thought about it, the more I realized that this information isn't something that people actively, regularly read about as I do.

I told her what I could during class, and then, that night, I went home and studied up on it even more. The next day, the down and dirty on high fructose corn syrup became our very first health tip.

It was then that we realized Hilliard Studio Method wasn't just a series of movements that we'd perfected; it was a lifestyle. We took very seriously our role in becoming experts for our clients, and we wanted to help them maximize the benefits of the workout with other ways to live more healthfully, more completely. There we were, the two of us in our twenties and fifties, and we were in the best shape of our lives and sharing it all with more than a thousand people every week.

At Hilliard Studio Method, we don't tell anybody exactly what to eat or when to eat it, because we all have our own lives and different dietary needs. What we do give, though, are guidelines, suggestions about how to fuel the body, what works for us, and what we have seen work for hundreds of clients of different ages and body types. We believe in *guidelines* not *restrictions*.

In the very same breath with which I just preached about not restricting yourself, I do have to give you my ultimate rule of three:

No sugar.

No sugar.

No sugar.

Refined sugar is the one thing I absolutely avoid in my food, and breaking yourself of your sugar habit will be the best thing you can do for yourself. I used to be addicted to sugar as a child and young adult as the majority of the population is. I don't know anyone who hasn't been addicted to sugar at some point in his or her life. But here's my nonscientific way of asking clients to come off it: cut it in half.

If you love your four cookies every night, for instance, then the next night, take two of those cookies and literally throw them in the trash. The next night, do the same thing, every night eating half until you're left actually not wanting the cookies in the first place! This same theory holds true for any food you may be struggling with and wishing you could just cut out of your diet. Whether you crave salty pretzels, white breads, creamy pastas, fried foods, sugary sports drinks, or coffee drinks, start with cutting your consumption of that food in half, and you may be surprised to find that you are actually satiated with less food, and your cravings will begin to diminish. It's a snowball effect. When you start cutting out the junk, you start to realize, *Wow, I can do this! I'm stronger than I thought I was.*

*P*rior to Hilliard Studio Method, I ran four times a week and dabbled in yoga and other fitness programs. However, as I approached forty, I could not lose weight—even if I exercised every day. I finally mustered up the courage to enroll in the Essential Method class. My first trainer, Amy Welton, introduced herself and encouraged me throughout the entire class. The other clients are incredibly welcoming and supportive as well. After completing my first class, I enrolled in the New Client Special. After completing the New Client Special I was hooked!

In addition to attending Hilliard Studio Method classes three times a week, I embraced Hilliard's nutritional philosophy, which includes no refined sugar. I used to feel constantly fatigued and dependent on a daily 3:00 p.m. treat to get me through the afternoon. Now, I am bounding with energy and am more productive. And I don't miss sugar!

I have been taking Hilliard Studio Method classes for two months. I am stronger and my clothes fit *much* better than before. I am so grateful to Hilliard Studio Method for helping me feel better in my forties than I did in my twenties or thirties.

–AMY RHYNE, AGE 43

The United States Department of Agriculture found an astonishing figure. The average American consumes five thousand tablespoons of refined sugar each year. That's the weight of an average American, approximately 150–170 pounds.[7] Wow! And don't be fooled; sugar lurks not just in the obvious sweets we think of as indulgences, such as candy bars and ice cream, but also in condiments, sauces, yogurt, soda, granola bars, cereal, frozen foods—the list goes on and on.

Even some of our fittest and cleanest-eating clients need reminders and tips from time to time about healthy eating, so I like to offer wellness seminars in the studio for some nutrition Q&A. Here's what one client took away, and I hope this chapter helps you gain some insight into my philosophy for a healthy lifestyle, which is not just a healthy diet but, rather, a balanced and holistic appreciation of your body and the fuel you choose to put in it.

Wow, what an impactful wellness seminar! I signed up because all things nutrition pique my interest, but I didn't expect to come away feeling so energized. I've been focused on eating real, clean food for years, but recently, I had become a bit bored with my food. As a result, some of my clean-eating habits had started to fray

---

7   Ellen Breslau, "9 Hidden Sources of Sugar in Your Diet," *The Huffington Post,* April 11, 2015, http://m.huffpost.com/us/entry/7020234.html.

at the edges (ahem, sugar). Since the seminar, I have made some adjustments to my diet and have noticed physical changes. More importantly though, I'm reengaged in the journey to incorporate even more whole, protein-packed foods into my diet because doing so makes me feel better. Liz gave us a bunch of great meal and snack ideas, but she also reinforced the importance of simply learning to love foods that our bodies love, and that just makes so much sense to me. Thanks for another hour well spent, albeit with no plank, at your studio!

–NIKKI CAMPO, AGE 37 —————————————————

EAT REAL FOOD

The thing is, if you limit yourself to diet restriction, if you deny yourself the things in life that make it enjoyable, then you're not living life to its fullest. That's just the simple truth. If you want to achieve a lifestyle of *joie de vivre*, you cannot constantly obsess over what to and what not to put into your body or scrutinize the choices you make. Instead, make a decision to be knowledgeable about the types of food you choose to eat. It won't take long to train your body and your brain to recognize real food as your friend and fake, processed food as your enemy. I

> It won't take long to train your body and your brain to recognize real food as your friend and fake, processed food as your enemy.

know that you can find a balance of healthy foods that are both interesting and delicious as well as good sources of fuel for your busy lifestyle. I always say you need to look at the foods you eat as either medicine or poison. I choose medicine!

Our favorite form of medicine comes in our signature Hilliard Studio Method smoothie, which we've also dubbed our "jet fuel." After fasting through the night, it's imperative that you fuel your body with protein, fiber, healthy fats, and vitamins and minerals. Those first things you put into your body every morning are more quickly absorbed because you have an empty stomach, so starting with a well-balanced meal is going to set you up for making better, healthier choices for the rest of the day.

HSM SIGNATURE SMOOTHIE

Ingredients:

¼ avocado

juice of ½ lime

1 cup organic mixed berries

2 scoops organic whey protein powder (rbh, grass-fed cow whey or goat whey)

1 scoop organic greens powder

1 scoop organic vitamin C powder

1 tbsp chia seeds

1 cup ice

2/3 cup coconut water

Blend ingredients, pop in a straw, and enjoy an energy-filled morning!

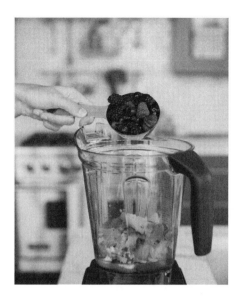

This is not your average smoothie. It's packed with twenty-seven grams of essential protein, twenty-three grams of fiber, and seven servings of organic, whole-food greens and vitamin C. This powerhouse combination of antioxidants, phytonutrients, vitamins, minerals, and healthy fats nourishes your muscles, organs, skin, and hair, making you feel satisfied and healthy all day long.

Benefits of the HSM Signature Smoothie

- *Avocado* is a nutrient-dense superfood loaded with heart-healthy, monounsaturated fatty acids, fiber, and potassium, plus nearly twenty vitamins and minerals. Avocado also lends a creamy texture to the smoothie, making it taste as good as a milkshake with none of the bad stuff!

- *Whey protein powder* is a naturally complete protein containing all of the essential amino acids to rebuild muscle tissue depleted through exercise. With protein, muscles recover faster, and lean muscle is built to speed up metabolism.

- *Organic greens powder* provides seven servings of green vegetables, enzymes, probiotics, and nutrients in one scoop.

- *Organic vitamin C powder* aids the absorption of greens; helps fight viruses; strengthens arteries, organs, and tissue; as well as promotes youthful skin through the promotion of collagen cell growth.

- *Chia seeds* are packed with omega-3s, protein, antioxidants, and fiber, which aids digestion and keep the body feeling fuller longer.

- *Coconut water* is full of electrolytes and potassium and is a great source of hydration and fuel for the body.

Other Superfoods You Can Add to Your Smoothie

- *Maca powder* is a superfood milled from the ancient maca root that is packed with vitamins, essential minerals, and amino acids. It is used to increase stamina, boost libido, promote hormonal balance, and combat fatigue.

- *Calcium Supplement* is a plant-based whole food is easily absorbed by the body and may reduce the risk of bone fractures, protect against certain cancers, help control blood pressure, and assist in weight management.

- *Fresh ginger and turmeric* are amazing roots that reduce inflammation, and research shows they can provide relief similar to that of ibuprofen.[8]

- *Herbs and other greens* add a fresh burst of flavor, vitamins, and phytonutrients to your smoothie. Pick from anything

---

8   Christopher D. Black, Matthew P. Herring, David J. Hurley, and Patrick J. O'Connor, "Ginger (*Zingiber officinale*) Reduces Muscle Pain Caused by Eccentric Exercise," The Journal of Pain, 11 (2010): 894–903, http://dx.doi.org/10.1016/j.jpain.2009.12.013.

you may have in your garden or from your local farmer's market. I personally love to add mint, basil, and parsley for an extra dose of flavorful greens.

Here's my formula for the rest of my meals and snacks:

- Choose local and organic foods.
- Eat lean protein.
- Load up on vegetables.
- Enjoy healthy fats.
- Choose fruit in its natural state.
- Beans are nature's diet pill.

CHOOSE LOCAL, EAT ORGANIC

I am adamant about eating food that has grown out of the ground as close to me as I can find, and so I buy organic groceries at local farmer's markets and retailers.

As explored in Michael Pollan's *In Defense of Food*, food products are processed echoes of whole foods created by food scientists hoping to engineer food better, and often more cheaply, than Mother Earth. Our bodies don't recognize these food products as food, and our systems get thrown for a loop. Our senses miss the "I'm full" signal and we overeat chemical-laden, processed foods.

There are three tips Pollan offers readers that have stuck with me every time I shop for groceries or reach for a snack:

1. *Eat simply*: Reach for foods that have grown out of the earth, and when choosing packaged items, look for those with five ingredients or fewer, and don't buy anything if you can't pronounce or read the name of an ingredient.

2. *Don't eat anything your great grandmother wouldn't recognize as food*: Let's just say your great-grandmother was born

sometime before or at the turn of the twentieth century. This would mean she wouldn't recognize anything preserved beyond a jar of pickles and certainly wouldn't consider eating anything in cellophane, shrink wrapped, or with a shelf life of over a week. Her bread would be baked fresh without preservatives, her eggs still in the shells, meat in the fridge or freezer, and her produce fresh.

3. *When shopping for groceries, stick to the perimeter of the store:* Just think. The perimeter has all of the natural foods: fruits and vegetables, fresh-baked bread, meat, seafood, dairy. Avoid the aisles lined with row after row of bags and boxes.

POWERFUL PROTEIN

When it comes to protein, I recommend a lot of it for everyone. Women, in general, don't get enough protein, because at an ideal sixty to a hundred grams a day, it's hard to do without overeating. Eating more protein doesn't mean you need to eat more overall. You need to omit overly processed, highly refined foods and incorporate plant and animal proteins into each meal. Animal-protein sources include meat, fish, dairy, and eggs, while vegetarian sources like beans, nuts, and legumes also deliver a good dose of protein.

Eating protein in the morning is especially important as it keeps your blood sugar steady for hours, which is why I enjoy my daily HSM Signature Smoothie made with organic whey protein. Organic Greek yogurt and eggs are other good sources of protein in the morning. Lean meat (organic and hormone free), fish (oily fish like wild salmon), or vegetarian protein with every meal will make a big difference in how fast you begin to see those six-pack abs!

At the same time, another wonderful benefit of protein is that it fills you up and helps prevent the dreaded sugar spike and fall. If you've ever started your day with a bowl of sugary cereal or a plate of pastries and doughnuts, you may have experienced how that blood-sugar spike affects you, making you feel sluggish and then hungry again not too long after your last meal. Set yourself up for a day of success with a good, healthy dose of nutrients and protein for breakfast.

I also eat organic whole, plain or Greek yogurt as a snack before heading out to dinner or a cocktail party. It keeps my hunger levels and blood sugar at bay and while the protein is filling, the healthy bacteria in the yogurt lines your gut with a dose of probiotics. Sometimes, I'll add a handful of fresh berries or some chia seeds for added flavor and crunch. This pre-party trick keeps you from over-indulging in the unhealthy choices found at most parties and keeps your stomach feeling better from the effects of alcohol.

VEGGIES: YOU CAN'T GET TOO MUCH

We all know we should eat our greens, and research says we should be consuming even more than we previously thought to reap the benefits. The old "five a day" might not be enough, reports the *Los Angeles Times*, suggesting that seven servings a day is necessary to reduce the risk of cancer, heart disease, and stroke.[9] This is why we love to have a scoop of organic greens in our smoothie every day. This single scoop is packed with seven servings of raw organic vegetables and gets your day off to a healthy start!

The more colors of the rainbow of vegetables you can get in your system every day, the better, but one of the best things you can

---

9   Mary MacVean, "'5-a-Day' might not be enough to ward off disease, scientists say," *Los Angeles Times,* April 1, 2014, http://www.latimes.com/science/sciencenow/la-sci-sn-fruit-vegetables-disease-20140401-story.html.

do for yourself is eat dark green, leafy veggies. The darker the green, the more essential vitamins and nutrients you're getting out of every bite, from protein to calcium, iron, fiber, folates, carotenoids, and vitamins C and K.

A team of North Carolina State University and Rutgers University researchers have discovered that certain plants, when ingested, produce steroids that "can increase lean body mass, the number of muscle fibers, and the endurance of the muscles themselves." Mustard greens, collards, broccoli, and kale may hold the "secret to stronger muscles, with none of the worrisome side effects of animal-derived steroids," the article explains. That's good news for all of us whether we're living a healthy lifestyle or recuperating from a debilitating disease. These natural plant-based steroids are also linked to antiaging![10]

DON'T BE AFRAID OF FAT

Are you serious? Yes, I am!

As explained in a Harvard Medical School online article, essential fatty acids (omega-3s and omega-6s) can actually boost your metabolism, control your blood sugar, and increase fat burning.[11]

The following foods are some of our "fat" foods:

Fish that's full of omega-3 fatty acids is healthy, such as salmon, albacore tuna, mackerel, and sardines. Watch out for mercury

---

10   "Newest Research: Greens Build Lean Muscle Mass and Increase Endurance," Hilliard Studio Method, January 13, 2013, http://www. hilliardstudiomethod.com/tips/newest-research-greens-build-lean-muscle-mass-and-increase-endurance?A=SearchResult&SearchID=701 9961&ObjectID=6099525&ObjectType=35.

11   "The truth about fats: the good, the bad, and the in-between," Harvard Health Publications, August 7, 2015, http://www.health. harvard.edu/staying-healthy/the-truth-about-fats-bad-and-good.

content, though, especially if you are pregnant. The general rule is the larger the fish, the higher the mercury content.

Avocados, nuts, chia seeds, and flaxseeds are nutrient dense, heart-healthy foods loaded with essential vitamins and fatty acids that not only make you feel great but do wonders for your skin, hair, and waistline. Full of omega-3 fatty acids, chia and flax seeds also contain protein and fiber, a perfect combination of nutrition, especially for those who choose a vegan or vegetarian diet.

Olive oil is heart healthy and maximizes nutrient absorption when you drizzle a bit of it over fresh vegetables. My all-time favorite way to use olive oil, though, is just like the iconic beauty Sophia Loren. She claims that olive oil is her body moisturizer of choice, and I've been following her advice for years!

I still remember when low-fat and no-fat cookies first came out in the early 1990s. As a model, I thought I could have as many of them as I wanted because there was no fat in them. My hair was crispy, thin, and falling out, and I felt sick from eating all that processed food! Full of chemicals and zero fat, I was starving even though I thought I was eating "healthy."

Stay away from "fat-free," "low-fat," and "reduced-fat" foods. Eat real butter, whole eggs, and whole yogurt. Eat food that you find locally and is raised without chemicals. If you're eating food out of a package, such as bacon or baloney, you're likely setting yourself up for an early death, not because of the fat content, mind you, but because of the carcinogens in all the chemicals used to preserve and process it.

Healthy fats are vital to your health. According to the Harvard Medical School article, "fat is a major source of energy. It helps you absorb some vitamins and minerals. Fat is needed to build cell membranes, the vital exterior of each cell, and the sheaths surrounding nerves. It is essential for blood clotting, muscle movement, and inflammation."[12] I'd say that's enough reason to enjoy a healthy dose of good fats in moderation.

AN APPLE A DAY

You may have read or heard that fruit has sugar and is therefore off-limits. It is true that not all fruits are created equal and can range in sugar content, so if you are watching more carefully what you are eating, you want to focus on the lower-sugar fruits. But the moral of the story is fruit contains natural sugars and is a wonderful source of fiber and many different antioxidants and vitamins.

I enjoy an organic apple every morning with my cup of green tea. Besides the fact that they're delicious, studies have found that apples can help lower cholesterol, manage diabetes, and prevent diseases such as cancer, cardiovascular disease, Alzheimer's disease, asthma, and osteoporosis.[13] The peel is not only a great source of insoluble fiber, which improves intestinal health, but it also contains an antioxidant called quercetin, which has been shown to reduce heart disease and inhibit the growth of tumors. The flesh of the apple contains a soluble fiber called pectin, which makes you feel full longer by slowing digestion and regulating blood-sugar levels. This sweet and satisfying fruit can stand in for your dessert craving at a mere eighty calories. So enjoy, and keep that doctor away!

---

12   Ibid.

13   "Why You Should Never Peel an Apple," *The Huffington Post,* February 19, 2014, http://www.huffingtonpost.com/2014/02/19/never-peel-apple_n_4791328.html.

HILLIARD STUDIO METHOD FAVORITE FRUITS

- blueberries
- raspberries
- blackberries
- strawberries
- pomegranates
- apples
- watermelons
- peaches
- oranges

DIET PILLS

No, not those! I'm talking about nature's little superfood: beans.

Beans make the perfect meal. High in fiber and protein and low in sugar, beans are filling, nutritious, easy to use, and affordable. They are a wonderful meat substitute, combat numerous diseases, and can be used in so many delicious recipes from soups to salads, but the most efficient way I use them is by boiling up a big batch on the weekend and serving myself a bowl with just a dash of salt whenever I'm feeling hungry. Black beans and lentils are some of my favorite legumes.

For a more complex and hearty meal, I combine black beans with quinoa, a grain that is naturally low in gluten, contains higher levels of protein than most grains, and—my favorite part—cooks in fifteen minutes! Its protein is complete, meaning it contains all the essential amino acids your body needs to function efficiently.

Here's an example of how I may incorporate all of these wonderful food sources into my day:

BREAKFAST

- organic green tea
- organic apple
- HSM Signature Smoothie

LUNCH

- oily fish such as salmon grilled on top of a green salad
- dressing: organic, cold-pressed olive oil, balsamic vinegar, salt, pepper, and the juice of a lemon

DINNER

- large salad of mixed greens and herbs topped with a variety of vegetables and fruits
- bowl of organic, homemade beans or grains such as lentils, black beans, or quinoa
- homemade popcorn, popped in coconut or olive oil, with salt, pepper, and a dash of garlic salt
- two glasses of red wine

SNACKS

- postworkout snack: handful of nuts or a Think Thin protein bar[14] and a Trilogy kombucha (favorite nuts include peanuts, almonds, walnuts, and cashews)
- afternoon snack: raw vegetables such as broccoli, cabbage, celery, and carrots with hummus.

---

14   Generally, packaged "energy" and "protein" bars are often loaded with sugar and are low in protein. When I need a quick and easy boost of protein with zero grams of sugar, the only bar I rely on is Think Thin Creamy Peanut Butter bars.

You probably noticed that I listed popcorn and wine with dinner. They are my *joie de vivre* foods. Wine absolutely turns into sugar in your body, but since it is the only added source of sugar in my diet and is something I can enjoy over a delicious meal, I'm going to enjoy a glass of wine, especially red wine, at the end of a long, hard day. I'm not saying you should go out and start drinking wine because of Hilliard Studio Method, but if you enjoy a glass of wine at night, we're not going to tell you that you can't have it. In fact, studies have shown that having a glass of wine a day may help preserve memory, prevent blood clots, boost good HDL cholesterol, burn a couple extra calories, guard against food poisoning, reduce the risk of certain cancers, boost bone mass, and reduce insulin resistance.[15] Whew!

I enjoy it with a bowl of popcorn, a snack food that offers more than just a satisfying crunch. As a whole grain, it boasts higher concentrations of fiber and fewer calories than cereals, chips, breads, and crackers. In a study, author Joe Vinson describes popcorn as "the perfect snack food," and the hull fragments, in particular, as "nutritional gold nuggets," because they contain high levels of antioxidants called polyphenols, which have been found to reduce the risk of cancer and heart disease.[16] Avoid packaged and processed popcorns, and don't slather your homemade popcorn with butter and salt.

15   Debra Gordon, "6 Reasons Why a Little Glass of Red Wine Each Day May Do You Good," Health, http://www.health.com/health/article/0,,20410287,00.html.

16   American Chemical Society (ACS), "Popcorn: The snack with even higher antioxidants levels than fruits and vegetables," ScienceDaily, March 25, 2012, https://www.sciencedaily.com/releases/2012/03/120325173008.htm.

DELICIOUS HSM POPCORN SNACK

Ingredients:

2 tbsp coconut oil

⅓ cup popcorn kernels

pinch of salt

seasoning of choice, such as:

- one teaspoon each of fresh thyme and rosemary
- one and a half teaspoons black truffle oil and three tablespoons freshly grated parmesan cheese
- one teaspoon each of smoked paprika and fresh parsley leaves
- two teaspoons fresh lemongrass stalk (inner part only) and two teaspoons lime zest

Method:

- Put the oil, popcorn, and pinch of salt in a large metal pot and cover.
- Turn the burner up to medium and shake the pot constantly.
- Remove from the heat and finish with your choice of seasonings.

I stay hydrated by drinking plenty of filtered water and a Kombucha (or three) a day. Kombucha tea contains billions of probiotics, antioxidants, B vitamins, and folic acid and is made from all-natural ingredients. With just sixty calories for a sixteen-ounce bottle of Synergy Kombucha tea, you will nourish and energize your body all day long!

Opt for these over diet soda and coffee drinks filled with milk products and no-calorie sweeteners, which not only leave you craving sweets but also make you bloated. Artificial sweeteners are difficult for your body to digest and actually cause you to gain weight instead of lose it.

THE UNSAVORY FACTS BEHIND ARTIFICIAL SWEETENERS

Dr. Hyman, MD, author of *The Blood Sugar Solution*, posits that insulin imbalance is the major cause of weight issues, diabetes, heart disease, cancer, dementia, and many other diseases. Craving sugar and refined carbohydrates and having low energy is not a natural state; it's a sign we are out of balance. While there are several key recommendations in his book, perhaps the simplest is dropping artificial sweeteners completely from your diet.

Dr. Hyman analyzed the data, and the results are not good for diet drinks.

"Those who consume diet drinks regularly have a 200 percent increased risk of weight gain, a 36 percent increased risk of prediabetes or metabolic syndrome, and a 67 percent increased risk of diabetes." And on top of that, people who drink two diet drinks a day have five times the increase in waist circumference as people who do not drink diet drinks. [17]

But perhaps the most shocking news was that in a bizarre study involving rats and cocaine, rats appeared to prefer artificial sweeteners to cocaine. And these rats had been programmed to be addicted to cocaine. To quote the author of the study, "The absolute preference for the taste of sweetness may lead to a re-ordering in the hierarchy of

---

17   Mark Hyman, MD, *The Blood Sugar Solution: The Ultra Healthy Program for Losing Weight, Preventing Disease, and Feeling Great Now!* (New York: Little, Brown and Company, 2012).

potentially addictive stimuli, with sweetened diets taking precedence over cocaine and possibly other drugs of abuse."[18]

Bottom line: It's time to give up artificial sweeteners such as stevia, aspartame, saccharine, xylitol, and the like, unless your goal is to gain weight, slow down your metabolism, and become an addict.

COFFEE OR TEA?

Stop putting nonsense in your coffee! Appreciate the natural flavors of your coffee beans and tea leaves. Enjoy it simply, without sugar or cream or artificial flavorings.

Clary and I reach for something in the morning that will pack a punch without the negative effects of sugar or high amounts of caffeine that other loaded coffee drinks may have. Green tea and specifically matcha tea, is a superfood that will get you set for your day by enhancing focus, naturally boosting your metabolism and providing you with an incredible dose of antioxidants. With its slow release of caffeine, matcha tea can be easily absorbed by the body and keep you energized throughout your day.

FUEL THE MACHINE

Our many different bodies are amazing miracle machines that are made up of cells and organs that function together to help us live. What we put into our bodies directly affects how well they function. Not only does food make us either look and feel good or bad, but it also causes our internal organs and our bloodstream to react either positively or negatively to the medicine or poison we choose to eat.

---

18   Mark Hyman, MD, "Why You Should Ditch Artificial Sweeteners," Dr. Hyman, http://drhyman.com/blog/2015/12/02/why-you-should-ditch-artificial-sweeteners/.

Eat healthy and delicious foods. Pay attention to what you eat and what is in your food. Then see how it makes you feel. Eating for Clary and me, and now many of our clients, is not about feeling deprived. It is about fueling ourselves to be able to do our workouts with energy, to feel good for the many things we want to do in a day, to live healthier, longer lives for our families and children. If you don't feel good after you eat, it's time to take a closer look at the changes you can make to give your body food that it can recognize and easily absorb and then use to promote healthy cell growth and decrease your risk for disease.

Unlike many HSMers, I didn't grow up a runner, dancer, or athlete. In fact, I did not really exercise at all for the first thirty-four years of life. I was naturally active as a child, playing in neighborhood creeks, woods, and swimming at the pool. Although my activity level lessened during my teen and young-adult years, I remained slim and coasted on those genes for years. Horror set in after having my second child when I realized my body wasn't bouncing back like it had after having my first child. I could no longer mindlessly eat the same foods as my husband and toddler without paying the price. The party was *over*. I was poofing up in my midsection—the area between my waist and knees . . . and it wasn't pretty. Clueless about nutrition and exercise yet too vain to "let myself go," I began working with a personal trainer who put me on a very high protein, heavy weight-lifting program. I also picked up tennis as a supplemental exercise/recreation activity.

Fast forward a few years and I was a beast . . . in more ways than one. Sure, I could do some serious lifting in the gym and overhead smashes on the courts, but I had bulked up from the intense lifting, felt toxic from the unbalanced diet (which included drinking lots of diet coke!) and was spending hours each week on the tennis courts. Outwardly, I appeared to be in great shape, but inwardly I was in a lot of pain and seeing an array of doctors, physical therapists, and masseurs for severe tendonitis, cortisone injections, acupuncture, and physical therapy. On top of that, I was spending *way* more time than I wanted in a competitive environment when I'm not even a competitive person! I was not returning to my former easygoing self, I was turning into a machine. None of it was resonating with me, and I was unhappy.

Luckily I found a new trainer who incorporated more cardio and got me off the heavy-protein regime. I leaned back out and felt much better. This transformation awoke me to the importance of being very intentional on how and with whom I exercised. At the time, I was the editor of a community magazine and was often coordinating with Clary. She always invited me to test out Hilliard Studio Method, and I promised I would if I ever took a break from tennis. I was definitely impressed by what I was hearing about the Method. And I personally knew several trainers and clients who were in amazing shape. Tennis wasn't doing that. My curiosity was piqued.

I finally decided to back off tennis and give Hilliard Studio Method a try. Confident in my fitness level, I thought it would be a cakewalk. The only thing that intimidated me as I strolled into that first Hilliard Studio Method class was having to bare my naked feet (not cute). About ten minutes in, my arms were toast, and I had dropped from eight- to five- to three-pound weights and was now using no weights and wondering if this was some kind of sick joke. The subsequent plank series was just plain brutal, and the spider and pretzel leg work had me begging for mercy. The final insult was the ab session.

Although I really hated that first class, I like a challenge, so I boldly purchased a ten pack. As I struggled through those ten classes, an amazing thing happened. The poofiness between my waist and thighs really toned up. My muscles became more defined, my thighs were slimmer than ever, and my abs were rock hard. My husband, family, and friends noticed as well. As I walked out after that tenth class, I knew I was part of something special. An efficient and goal-oriented person, it just made sense—great results, less time. Added perks included great upbeat music, a beautiful studio, and knowledgable, encouraging trainers.

I've been doing Hilliard Studio Method for almost two years now and have yet to see a chiropractor or orthopedist. The wonderful Hilliard Studio Method trainers constantly instruct me on proper form and how to modify if needed, as well as stress the importance of listening to my body. I also *love* the positive and encouraging synergy of the classes—a welcome change from the competitive, often negative, energy of competitive sports. And the efficiency can't be beat. In one hour, *all* areas of the body are addressed and toned. I love the challenge and the results. I look forward to the weekly

Hilliard Studio Method newsletter for the latest tips on health, nutrition, fitness, and fashion. On top of all that, I especially appreciate Hilliard Studio Method's commitment to good causes and giving back to the community.

I still tucker out toward the end of biceps, silently suffer my way through plank, and beg for mercy during fold over, but I'll keep going, keep trying to master it and keep reaping the benefits of the Hilliard Studio Method program.

–CINDY MARKEY, AGE 51 ————————————————————

It's never too late to make choices that help you look and feel healthy, powerful, and strong. Take care of your body from the inside out, and you will find a joy that I hope will last a very long lifetime.

6 YOU ARE POWERFUL

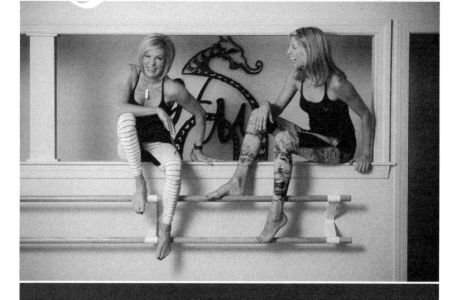

CHAPTER 6:
YOU ARE POWERFUL

I love the power of Nike's mission statement that simply says, "If you have a body, you are an athlete."

The athletes that make up the trainers and clients at Hilliard Studio Method come from all walks of life and are all different sizes, shapes, and ages. I have written about how joy is a thread throughout my life and a pathway to my authentic self. My greatest joy in getting to know my employees and our clients is learning about their journeys. I have the privilege of getting to know their hardships, heartaches, and disappointments as well as their successes, achievements, and celebrations. I find joy in seeing clients become a little stronger each day. I understand the mental, emotional, and physical strength it takes for them to get up and commit to an hour of our workout, to make health a priority, to believe that they can push a little harder on their mat and therefore push a little harder in all aspects of their lives to become more powerful. Every time we hit a side plank, I remind the clients to look above my head on the wall at our "Be Powerful" sign. I tell them to read it and to know it, because they are.

*I*n October 2010, I became a "living" statistic that no one should want to become; I survived a deadly infection to my body commonly called the "flesh-eating bacteria." The infection came from a small cut to the top of my left foot, when I dropped a computer on it, and resulted in the amputation of that same leg below the knee.

Much has happened since that fateful day nearly three years ago. I initially remember having some very long days, just learning how to walk again, how to care for my two young boys, and how to do everyday things in a different way, including bathing myself. Today, I do not take anything for granted, and I especially have developed a stronger appreciation for fitness and a healthy lifestyle. Above all, individuals who go through a traumatic injury such as amputation are more likely to become sedentary in their lifestyles. This habit can create further complications such as diabetes, depression, and obesity and makes the individual even more of a health-care burden on themselves and loved ones.

Today, I embrace healthy activity more than ever. Since starting Hilliard Studio Method, my core and upper body have greatly gained more muscle strength that I have not been able to accomplish in other workout classes. In addition, isolating the muscles and being able to feel the burn has been effective in gaining form in my upper left leg. I am seeing a more balanced appearance in muscle tone between my amputated (left) leg and my sound (right) leg. This balance, both metaphorically and physically, under the watchful care of the Hilliard trainers, has made me a much more whole person.

If you're having a bad day and don't think you can fit Hilliard into your lifestyle, think of the challenges I face. Thank you, Liz, for creating this incredible workout and for making me feel "complete" again!

–JANELLE LENHART, AGE 42

One of our clients, a breast-cancer survivor in her midsixties, recently participated in a local Dancing with the Stars competition in support of a local breast-cancer charity. She attended class regularly to prepare her body for the physical demands of the competition and worked with determination for several months. Although she did not win the competition, she did find the strength to step outside her comfort zone and surprise herself with some newfound dance moves, muscle tone, and stamina, and it was all for a good cause. What an inspiration! But one of the things I considered so meaningful about her journey was when she said to Clary, "A Hilliard Studio Method workout for me is like being in Latin class and I'm speaking pig Latin, but no one is laughing at me!" I was thrilled to hear this sentiment: that she felt supported even if she didn't always feel confident in what she was doing. When you start to move forward, even if it's just baby steps, you begin to see how far you can go, and you begin to discover your power. That power already exists in you, and at Hilliard Studio Method we just remind you that it's there.

I admit I remember walking into my first class and thinking, *I got this!* But within the first ten minutes of class, I realized I did not have it, but I wanted it. What is it? These ladies are balancing on one leg doing overhead presses. There is a reason behind every-thing they do. I work on my mind/body connection, build core strength, and with each class, gain the confidence that one day I can say "I really do have it!" And when something throws that off schedule, I honestly get a bit grumpy and I don't feel right. My body needs this workout; it craves this workout. It has become so much more than just working out for me. As a mom of two small children, it is my break, my quiet time, my therapy! I look forward to walking through the door at Hilliard Studio Method because each time I show up, I continue to build the healthiest, strongest version of me possible. I love how strong I feel, how I can crank out a few sets of push-ups, no problem. And toned abs after children. Give me more!

Now, when I conquer the whole ten-minute plank series without breaking, I will feel like I have conquered the world. Baby steps . . .

Liz and Clary really have this figured out. It is no wonder that so many people I come in contact with have heard great things about Hilliard Studio Method. I want to shout it from the rooftops that every woman needs this workout. It is one of the most challenging workouts you can do, but even the most beginner of students can walk through the door and accomplish it in some capacity. That's the beauty of it.

–NATALIE PULVER, AGE 36 ————————————

One of our teachers started working for us when she was just twenty-six years old. She was dating a man whom she thought she was going to marry. However, things started going south, and she made the difficult and emotional decision to walk away from the relationship. She was devastated but knew she had made the right decision. Fast-forward a few years, and now she's recently married to her perfect match. Clary and I both went to her engagement party, and while we were there, she stopped us and said, "Liz, I just have to tell you that I'll never forget the day you grabbed my arm just after a class and said, 'Walk away from that guy and don't look back.' You said it with such strength and power, and I knew you were right. I was afraid, but I did it. And I can't thank you enough because I was able to leave him and now I'm marrying this amazing guy!"

Each of us has a story. It may be an amazing one of rising from nothing or simply a moment in which we acknowledge and embrace our own strength. No matter where you are in life, it's important to understand your own strength. You have the power to take that step, whether it's away from something negative or toward something better, or both! And the more you feel supported, the more strength and support you have to give. When you are your authentic self and can release that energy into the world around you, you can spark the power and passion in others. That empowerment, of women supporting women, can't be underestimated. It's important at every stage in life, and it's our goal to give that power to clients every time they walk in our door.

Everyone—and I mean *everyone*—finds our workouts challenging. I would put my Method up against any workout out there. But in having that reputation, it also makes it difficult for some people just to walk in the door. So we celebrate those who do and teach them with a constant stream of encouragement, a promise that they can do it until they believe they can. Many times, people don't understand why they love coming to Hilliard Studio Method so much.

They can point out certain aspects they enjoy, but so many of them say to us, "Why do I love it? I cannot *not* be here." And that's the magic of "Be Powerful." They come into our physical space for a solid hour where we support and challenge their different levels of fitness with an even hand until at the end of class they simply *feel better*. They feel stronger, they stand taller, and they start to feel mentally and emotionally stronger as well, making "Be Powerful" not just about a push-up but also about a way of life.

> "Why do I love it? I cannot *not* be here." And that's the magic of "Be Powerful."

When you find yourself amid the chaos of life, your friends and family can love and support you, but no one can find your power but you. That is why I began this story with the quote about the difference between a warrior and an ordinary man. We are not the result of what happens to us but the result of how we respond to life's challenges.

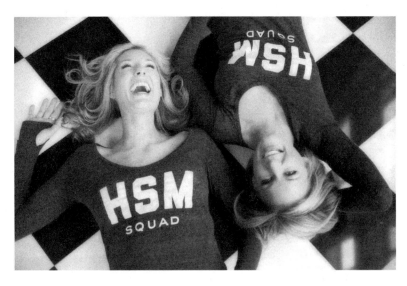

MORE THAN A WORKOUT–IT'S A WAY OF LIFE

In the end, being powerful is simply accepting who you are at your most basic level. It's not about getting to the end; it's about your journey and finally accepting your darkness (weakness) along with your light (strength) to become your authentic self, your most powerful version of you. Being powerful is claiming who you are and responding to that legitimately and honestly and being able to stand up in the presence of whatever life has handed you in that moment and knowing that you have the strength to step forward. You have that power in you, but it's up to you to believe you are worthy.

I come from a family of chiropractors, so health has played an important role in my life, but less than a year ago, I began to struggle. I became frustrated that I hadn't found a method of exercise I was truly passionate about. I started to lose motivation to go to the gym and blamed it on working nine to five. My lack of motivation kept me from pushing myself, and I developed what I call an unhealthy mentality. I stopped exercising, stopped eating nutritional foods, and wallowed in my own negativity. I felt defeated. I lost sight of my own self-image and became unhappy with my appearance. I had let my own mind talk me into quitting, and I knew I had to change.

It wasn't until I literally started to feel sick and tired–sick of feeling exhausted at work and tired of hearing my own negative thoughts that a dear friend and long-time "HSM groupie" encouraged me to try it out. My first class was amazing and challenging. From the warm welcome I received to the energy the class brought, I knew it was for me. I made a commitment thereafter that I would never let myself get to the place I was at before. I now have more energy, confidence, and strength. Through Hilliard Studio Method, I learned that "change doesn't come from your comfort zone; it comes from your edge." I've also learned that class doesn't get easier, but I get stronger! The trainers ensure proper form and safety (which my chiropractors appreciate) and make each class unique and fun. That is what keeps me coming back! Thanks to Hilliard Studio Method, I have been brought back to good health, both mentally and physically!

–SARA SMITH, AGE 26

So what's next? You are now equipped with the knowledge and reasons *why* Hilliard Studio Method is the choice of so many women and how it has changed lives—how it has empowered, strengthened, and transformed bodies and minds.

When you decide to intently start on the path to your complete well-being, the path to your healthy lifestyle, the instructors and community at Hilliard Studio Method are here to support, strengthen, and challenge you in all the best ways. This is a place where you can find your strength and push your body to your edge.

What began as a quest to simply know everything there was to know about Pilates because it ignited a fire inside me turned out to be the reason why I was able to create a Method that not only brought Clary and me together but also created a community of empowerment.

I created a Method, and we created a business that defines our *joie de vivre* and embraces the hardships as a part of the process—the perfect balance. We keep moving forward, and we keep evolving, knowing that at any moment life can change but that our love and joy will overcome it.

"When you have come to the edge
of all the light you know
And are about to step off into the
darkness of the unknown,
One of two things will happen, there will
be something solid to stand on
Or you will be taught to fly."

–Barbara Winter

Step forward. Be Powerful.
—Liz

HILLIARD STUDIO METHOD
CHISELED ARMS ROUTINE

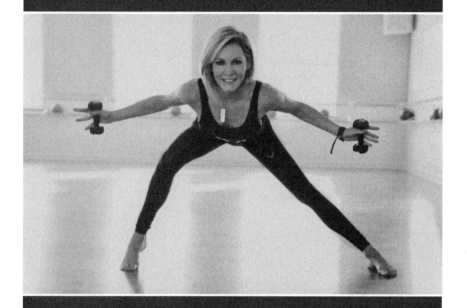

BONUS CHAPTER:
HILLIARD STUDIO METHOD CHISELED ARMS ROUTINE

*For this and many more Hilliard Studio Method workouts, visit **hilliardstudiomethod.com** to purchase DVDs or download a full selection of workouts to help you find your healthiest, most powerful self!*

Ready to sculpt your upper body like never before, burn some calories, rev up your metabolism, and reshape your body? In this chapter, we're going to give you a taste of what a quick, twenty-minute Hilliard Studio Method routine might look like. Keep in mind that no class is the same, including this intermediate workout. Every move can have dozens of variations. So don't expect to see this exact workout on a visit to Hilliard Studio Method. Muscle confusion is one of the secrets to the Method sauce, and we like to keep your mind and body guessing!

As with any class, we encourage you to have a towel and water bottle handy because we are going to sweat! Are you ready? Then let's get started with what we like to call the Hilliard Studio Method chiseled arms routine.

What you'll need: eight-pound weights, three-pound weights, no shoes, and a whole lot of spirit!

Start by picking up your eight-pound weights, but if you are brand-new to exercise or rehabbing an injury, then I suggest starting with a lighter weight such as six, five, or three pounds. Keep in mind, however, that to really change your body, the heaviest set of weights you can safely use is the one you want to choose

In class, I suggest that our clients have a buffet of weights (several different sizes) ready to use. That way they can drop down to a lighter weight if they are struggling and then go back to the heavy weights when they're ready. You can do the same at home, but remember the goal is to safely find your edge!

FIND YOUR CORE

In order for a move to be Hilliard Studio Method approved, it must be 100 percent efficient and equally 100 percent safe. I can control the moves, but you have to control your body, especially when working out on your own. And the sure-fire way to control your body is to find your core connection. Why?

1. It protects your back.
2. It strengthens your abdominals and back while you're working other muscle groups.
3. It increases the efficiency of the workout.

Holding your heavy weights, position your feet under your sitz bones, the middle part of your glutes, and then slightly bend your knees.

Take a deep breath in through your nose and bring your shoulders up to your ears.

Exhale through your mouth and drop your shoulders down your back as you open your chest and keep your chin parallel to the floor.

Maintain this good posture and repeat another deep breath, this time paying attention to what your abdominals do. As you blow out, pull your belly button in deeply as you fight the urge to squeeze your booty muscles. On the third round of breaths, stand tall, pull your belly in, and finally, pull in the sides of your waist by your rib cage in and down. Throughout these exercises, continue moving your breath and your abdominal muscles just like this. It may help you to visualize your core gently zipped up in a jacket.

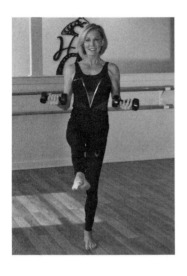

STANDING BICEP CURLS

To warm up, we start with a simple standing bicep curl. Bend your elbows, bringing your heavy weights up toward your shoulders, and then extend them down by your sides. Keep your arms slightly ahead of you and by your sides, being aware to never lock your elbows or sling your weights. If you are slinging, it's a sign you need to use lighter weights to start. But no worries. We all have to start somewhere! Repeat fifteen curls, and if you've already forgotten about your core, it's time to pull it back in.

Adding balance to your curls, bring your right knee up to hip level. As you curl your arms up, extend your leg out in a kick as straight as you can get it. Bend the knee back to its starting position as you extend your arms from the curl. Complete fifteen reps, knowing you can always keep both feet on the ground. For the final challenge here, hold the leg straight, bend your arms ninety degrees, and hold a half curl. Pulse your arms and leg up one inch ten times.

We're still in the biceps, but the next stop is Texas!

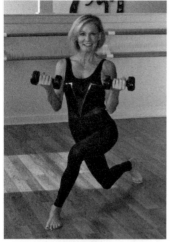

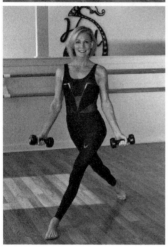

TEXAS CURTSY BICEP CURLS

This curtsy move is great for the lower body and waist and challenges the core by making the upper and lower body work at the same time. While this exercise can be used to engage all of the primary muscle groups, it's particularly challenging for the glutes because they're kept in constant tension, strengthening and sculpting these muscles as we move the body straight up and down like an elevator.

With your core engaged, take your right leg and sweep it behind the left on a diagonal in a deep curtsy, keeping both feet facing forward and your front left knee lined up directly over your left toes. Make sure your feet are far apart to the point where you almost can't feel your thighs touch. Twist through your torso so that both shoulders are squared forward to engage the obliques or side waist muscles.

Bend your front knee in half until your hip drops as low as your knee. At the same time, deeply bend your back knee until it almost touches the floor. You want to go as low as you can to work your gluteal muscles. Keep your core engaged to make sure your back feels comfortable and strong. Have you ever seen a debutante curtsy? They get low! And that's what we're going to do now.

Moving down and up, again like an elevator, bend your knees and curl your arms up, and as you lift out of the curtsy, extend your arms down. Don't come all the way out of the curtsy, though. You want to maintain contraction in the gluteal muscles and keep the breath controlled as you exhale on the exertion of the curtsy and the bicep curl.

Complete fifteen of these full-range Texas curtsy bicep curls, and on the last one, hold low. Next, complete fifteen pulses just as you did in standing bicep curls. Staying low in your curtsy and, if you can, lifting your left front heel to advance it, pulse your hips down an inch and your arms up an inch at the same time. Your glutes are probably screaming for you to stand right now. So make sure your front heel is down and your core pulled in to come to standing.

Time to work your left leg with the same moves—I know—at least we only have two legs!

- fifteen standing bicep curls + pulses
- fifteen standing bicep curls + kicks and pulses
- fifteen Texas curtsy curls + pulses

You'll be able to tell by now if you need to pick up heavier weights or drop down to lighter weights. You should be feeling the heat, but we have a few moves left, so stick with it!

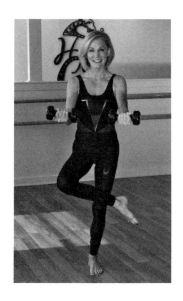

CONCENTRATION

This is a trick we do at Hilliard Studio Method because it is a signature mind/body move. Believe me, there's a lot of wiggling and starting over for our clients on this one!

From your standing, core-connected position, bend your right leg into a figure-four shape by crossing your right ankle over your left thigh. Bend your standing left leg, slightly

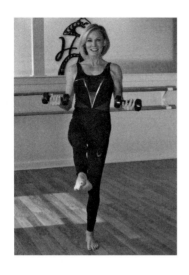

hinge forward from the hips, and reach your arms forward and away from your body, palms facing the ceiling as if you were serving a platter. Look in a mirror if possible. Are your shoulders curved and rounding forward? If so, open your chest back up and flatten your back before moving to the fun part.

Bring your arms back to your sides, and at the same time, kick your right leg so that it's straight out from your hip and come to standing. Bend the right leg to make a figure four again, reach the arms forward, and then kick and squeeze. You did it! This move is challenging on both a fast and slow beat, and working multiple body parts in different directions has earned the move its name. Work up to fifteen reps on each leg to really get some bang for your buck. Your last set of biceps is coming up!

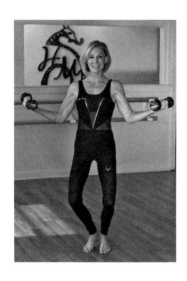

NARROW V BICEP CURLS

Put your heels together, toes apart at forty-five-degree angles similar to the first position in ballet. Lift your heels up about an inch off the floor, and bend at the knees as though your back is sliding down an imaginary wall until your legs form a diamond shape. We love how quickly your quadriceps (thigh muscles) are going to feel this one!

For the first set, open your arms wide to forty-five-degree angles. Hold as low as you can in your legs and complete fifteen curls.

Next, bring your arms back in front of your body, but don't stand up yet! In fact, see if you can drop it one more inch! Complete ten curls.

Finally, find your power and drop it one inch lower than last time. With your arms bent halfway at ninety degrees, complete ten final pulses, only moving an inch in your arms and legs. As you pulse your hips down, your arms pulse up.

You did it—awesome job! Take a break by bringing your weights to your chest. You've just worked your biceps and what we call our Popeye muscles. You know the image of Popeye flexing his arm with that spinach can by his side? Well, we love spinach, but it won't give you the definition that Hilliard Studio Method chiseled arms can.

Next up, we work your "coconut muscles" (medial deltoids), which are the tops of your shoulders. Pressing heavy weights overhead is one of the most important times you need to stay aware of your form, your posture, and your core, so reset and let's get started.

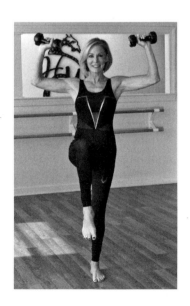

OVERHEAD PRESS

With a slight bend of the knees and a nice, long spine, press your arms overhead. They should be slightly in front of your body so when you glance up you can see the weights in your peripheral vision as you press the weights overhead. Keep your ribs and belly zipped up and don't lean back. Bend the elbows, bringing them down with control to shoulder height.

That is one rep. Continue to breathe through eight presses and then add a controlled kick. Just like the bicep-curl kick, bring your right leg up to hip level. Perform an overhead press with a kick, and return to the starting position eight times. Hold the leg extended, keep the elbows bent, and give it a set of one-inch pulses before we take it back to curtsy.

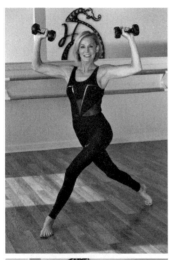

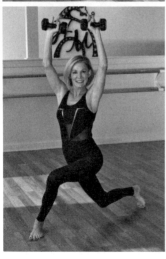

TEXAS CURTSY OVERHEAD PRESS

This lower-body move is exactly the same curtsy you performed during the biceps exercise. So take your right foot behind your left and get low. Press your arms overhead as you curtsy, and then bend the elbows no lower than shoulder height as you lift the legs. Just as before, keep your torso facing forward and pull in through your core. You will probably have to remind yourself to breathe here, and I promise it will help! You have eight reps to do, and I know you can do it!

One side left. If you need to bring the weights to your chest, go for it. As you get stronger and are able to keep your arms lifted throughout this series, you are going to feel the added cardio benefits!

- eight standing overhead presses
- eight standing overhead presses + kicks
- eight Texas curtsy overhead presses

And for the grand finale, find your original standing position and give me your best eight overhead presses. Nothing fancy but a whole lot of hard work! Well done!

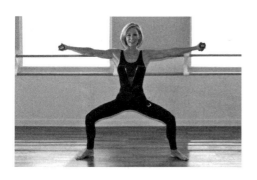

WIDE SECOND IRON CROSS DELTOID WORK

Most gymnasts know what iron cross means. It's an incredible position in which both arms extend out to a perfect T and hold hanging rings as the body holds stillness in the air. I like to remind clients that we're lucky to have our feet on the floor for this one!

In this move, you're going to mimic an iron cross hold with your arms. Hold a pair of three-pound weights in each hand and extend them to a T with palms facing the floor.

Walk your legs out much wider than your hips, turning your toes out again in forty-five-degree angles and bend at the knees with the goal of dropping the hips until the legs are parallel to the floor. You may have tighter hips or weaker knees, and if so, you will stay in a higher position, knowing each time you work here, you are giving your muscles a gentle stretch as you strengthen them. Reach the crown of your head to the ceiling to elongate through the spine, and zip up the imaginary jacket around your torso.

With arms extended, perform a small pulse. Hips move down one inch and arms move up an inch at a steady beat. Complete fifteen reps.

Even though you're holding three-pound weights, your arms probably feel as if they're holding fifteen or twenty pounds each after the heavy weight work you just finished. So if it becomes too much, go ahead and put the weights down and make a fist with your hands so you are still working in contraction and not just flailing about.

For your next move, just flip your palms to face behind you so that your pinky fingers face the ceiling and your thumbs face the floor. As usual, I'm going to challenge you to drop your hips one inch lower. You don't know how strong you are until you try! When you are working multiple muscle groups, one muscle group often forgets its job as your brain focuses on another.

From here, gently press your arms back to open the front of your chest and, at the same time, press your thighs back as well. This is a three-part move. Press your arms back a tiny inch, then another, then a final press back, and hold. Say, "Press, press, squeeze," as you complete this ten times.

Rotate your palms back to the floor for another set of ten pulses. For the last move, you actually won't move. Keep your arms still and your hips low, and to really challenge yourself, see if you can lift your heels off the floor and feel your legs shake for a final hold. Don't speed count! Try "One Mississippi, two Mississippi . . ." until you can hold for ten seconds.

THE FAT-BURNING ZONE

At this point, your heart rate is elevated and you may be sweating. This is some serious cardio, and we're working your heart rate in the fat-burning zone. This is one of the key reasons Hilliard Studio Method works so well.

Don't be fooled! While many equate cardio with sweating bullets and huffing and puffing until you're completely out of breath, actually elevating your heart rate to half of its maximum rate the way we do at Hilliard Studio Method is the best way to sculpt muscles and burn fat! We are safely pushing you to your edge without putting undue pressure on your joints. In fact, the safe, low-impact movements here and in all of our workouts promote strength in your joints, allowing your body to tone up but also work for you for a long time to come! Challenge yourself, but always listen to your body if it's telling you it's time for a break.

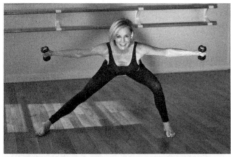
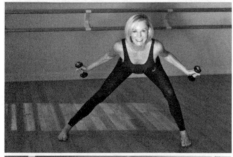
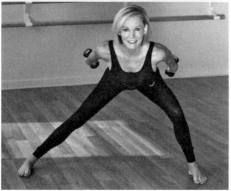

SPEED SKATER POSITION

We call this the speed skater position because you mimic Apollo Ohno, whipping around a track, hinged nice and low, with your weight shifted into one leg and the other leg extended.

By hinging forward and holding our arms out, we begin to work the posterior, or back side, of the shoulder muscles as opposed to the medial, or top part, of the deltoids we worked previously. And speaking of "posterior," your glutes will definitely feel it in this position, not to mention your core is fully engaged to keep you here.

To begin from a wide second iron cross, bring your weights to your chest, breathe, roll your shoulders back, and turn your toes forward. Then hinge forward with a flat back, and lunge into your right leg by bending your knee and shifting your weight to your right hip as you drive your hips back as if you're sitting in a chair, and lengthen through the inner thigh of your straight left leg. Keeping your elbows by your side, swing your arms out wide until your palms face forward as though you're flying. Give your arms a little press back and squeeze between your shoulder blades. I explain the squeeze as though you have a pencil between your shoulders blades and you don't want to let it drop.

Begin to press back ten times as you hold stillness in your lower body. Then intensify with a back, back squeeze motion on a one-two-three count. On the final press, squeeze extra hard.

Your next challenge will be to stay in the lower-body speed skater position as we move to the triceps muscles on the back of your arms. I know how it's burning now; you're almost there!

Bring your arms back to your chest and then extend them back behind you like a snow skier launching from a takeoff ramp. Your knuckles will be facing out and your palms facing in as you begin to pulse your arms just an inch at a time toward the ceiling.

Maintain your core connection and pulse your arms straight up fifteen times. On the last pulse, hold your arms up as high as you can for three, two, one!

Fantastic! Let's reset and do the other side. Hinge into your left side speed skater lunge and complete the same moves again:

- ten posterior delts press backs
- ten posterior delts back, back, squeeze, and hold
- fifteen triceps lifts and hold

There are so many muscles around your spine working while you do this move! And don't forget to thank those gluteal and core muscles that are working hard to keep you in this position.

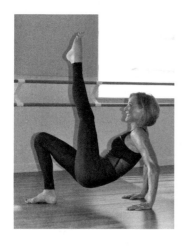

TRICEPS DANCING

Now you get to put those weights down and have a seat on the floor, but don't be fooled, this too will make you sweat and shake! We call this triceps dancing because we add some flair to the legs as we fire into the triceps.

Have a seat with your knees bent, feet flat. Place your hands on the floor behind you underneath your shoulders with your fingers facing forward. Lift your hips high off the floor into a reverse bridge as you scoop your belly toward your spine. Lift out of the shoulders with an open chest.

Lift your right leg and cross your right ankle over your left knee. Bend your elbows deeply, and as you press away from the floor, kick your leg in the air like a can-can dancer. Your hips will lower, but make sure your arms are doing the work. Bend and extend the arms and legs together for ten reps. Just as you are contracting through the arms, shoot energy through your leg and out of your toe as it extends.

Hold the last one with your arms straight and your leg extended in the air. Bend your elbows just a couple of inches, and then pulse up an inch ten times. You can always keep both feet on the floor for this. The primary work is in the backs of the arms, but we always like to give our moves, minds, and bodies an added challenge whenever we can!

Slowly lower your extended right leg down and hover it over the floor. As you bend and press the arms, move the right leg out an inch and back in an inch. This is hard work, not only on your arms and core but now through the back of your left supporting hamstring. Make sure to keep those hips level and off the floor as you repeat ten outs and ins with the triceps press.

As you bring your right leg back to the floor beside the left to repeat on the other side, see if you can keep your hip lifts, but take a break if you need it. You're halfway there.

- ten can-can dancer kicks
- ten can-can dancer pulses
- ten hover outs and ins

Your arms are almost chiseled. Here's your final move!

With both feet flat and both knees bent, bend your elbows in half and pulse down an inch ten times and then back up one inch ten times.

That's it, you did it!

STRETCH!

Now go ahead, sit back down, and move into a comfortable cross-legged position.

Reach your right arm to the ceiling, bend your elbow in half, and reach your fingertips down your back. Gently press the elbow with your left hand to give your triceps a deeper stretch. Release and sweep your right arm in front of your chest, extending it out with energy. Use your opposite arm to hug it toward your body to give your shoulders a gentle stretch. Turn your gaze over the shoulder to the right as you sit tall. Repeat both stretches with your left arm.

To open your chest, clasp your hands behind your back, extending the arms as straight and high as possible as you gently lift your chin. Hold for a round of breath, and then reverse the stretch, clasping your hands together in front of your body. Flip your palms away from you, tuck your chin to your chest, and curve through your spine as you take your gaze to your belly button.

Ending by focusing on your core, place your hands on your thighs, roll your shoulders down your back, breathe in deeply, and as you exhale, draw your belly button in and your ribs in and down.

Well done! You have just chiseled and sculpted your arms with this signature Hilliard Studio Method short workout.

ACKNOWLEDGMENTS

I recently read a quote, "find your tribe and love them hard." When I created this workout for my daughter Clary, I had no idea it would become a lifestyle for us both and a cornerstone to my health and longevity as well as thousands of others. I'm keenly aware of the love and support it takes of some very important people in my life who have embraced my passion and keep inspiring me to stay fearless, keep creating and share my knowledge with others—my Tribe. Inspiration greets me every single day I walk into my "happy place"-Hilliard Studio Method. It's a place of joy, community, strength, and love. It's powerful.

Of course, I must first acknowledge Clary: my joy, inspiration, daughter, and best friend. Simply put, Hilliard Studio Method would not be what it is today without her. I wouldn't be me without her.

My eternal thanks go to my husband Aubrey. He is my true love, strong arm of support, and ceaseless friend who encourages me to never fit the mold and always be myself. He keeps me laughing and gets full credit for some of my favorite sayings and chapter titles— *Stronger Than Train Smoke* and *Going through Hell in Gasoline Drawers*—and has never once criticized me for not knowing where the grocery store is!

To Robert Gray; smart, patient, endlessly supportive, a wonderful husband to Clary and father to my grandchildren. I couldn't ask for a better son-in-law.

To my granddaughter Aubrey and grandson Cameron, for keeping me exceedingly joyful and in love with every new day!

My Tribe members who remind me to "Be Powerful" every day include:

Lee Kennelly, who knows my heart and soul like no one else and spent countless hours encouraging me through the tears and fears of my own inadequacies to keep writing this book and share the joy that is my truest self. To empower another is to truly "Be Powerful." Thank you dear friend.

Carrie Deaton, who wears her power like a seven-foot warrior woman in a deceivingly petite frame. She empowers me by keeping my feet to the fire and my business running on track in the face of daily chaos.

Leah Williams, who is my self-professed consigliere, video producer, friend, and organizer extraordinaire. Leah announced to me after I had hired her that she had actually accomplished a non-hostile takeover of HSM. If I said anymore, that would be "too many words."

Lindsay Rothrock, calm, collected, smart and capable at such a young age. So proud to have her on my team!

Meg Morrison Peebles, my friend and part of the family from day one. She makes every party, every trip and every day more fun, while setting the HSM bar high with her extraordinary work and professionalism.

Jennifer Shelton and Amy Welton, good friends, great trainers and part of this amazing HSM team from the very beginning. Thank you!

Arthur Pulley, who joined us as our Head Coach at HSM | Core on a leap of faith when we opened our second business. His motivation and energy are endless and enthusiasm contagious!

A world of thanks to all of the trainers at Hilliard Studio Method and all of the coaches at HSM | Core who inspire me every day by embracing the essence of "Be Powerful," and inspire each person who walks through our doors to find his or her most powerful self: Lee Kennelly, Meg Peebles, Jennifer Shelton, Amy Welton, Madison Kennedy, Tara Hughes, Michlene Healy, Sara Gray, Elizabeth McNabb, Lauren Bolshakov, Donna Short, Brittany Williams, Rebecca Fallon, Arthur Pulley, Dayron Booth, Jerome Touchstone, Kristi Kemp, Andrea Kiely, Mary Margaret Allen, Francie Rudolph.

And, of course, many thanks to those amazing women who staff our front desk, answer endless questions and ease the anxiety of our first time clients including: Ashley Walker, Abbey Leitner, Grace Herrin, Addison Abee, Molly Lando, Adair Carpenter, Preston Fogartie.

To my sister, Wallis, who always believed in me when no else did, least of all myself, and continues to think everything I touch is magic.

To my brother, Pete, who kept me honest, safe, laughing, and ready to take a punch! As my first self-appointed coach he taught me the fine skills of perfecting my jump shot and drive the lane regardless of the 6-foot girl waiting to pummel me. His love is unspoken and unbreakable.

To my dad, who left me with the most powerful message of all, noblesse oblige; that it was my duty to walk humbly through the world and honor people from all walks of life and treat them in equal measure. His strength and tenderness are a part of me, and for that I am forever grateful.

To my mom, the most powerful woman I have ever known. She was brilliant, strong and looked every situation bravely in the eye. No one could ask for a better role model than that. With grace, determination and love she led me to find my power.

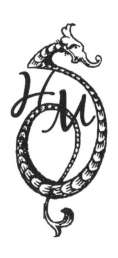